"Prostate cancer is a major men's health problem. Over the past several years the proportion of cases with early localized disease has increased dramatically in parallel to questions regarding the optimal management of these patients. Today, perhaps more than ever, men diagnosed with prostate cancer face the frustrating challenges around management decisions of their disease. This books offers a concise, up-to-date and balanced discussion of most critical aspects involved in this process in a very easy-to-read format."

Mario A. Eisenberger, MD
R. Dale Hughes Professor of Oncology and Urology
Sidney Kimmel Comprehensive Cancer Center
The Johns Hopkins University
Baltimore, MD

"A concise, contemporary, comprehensive guide for men and their families who are dealing with a diagnosis of prostate cancer. Dr. Burnett, an international expert, brings the most important questions to the forefront with simple, straightforward answers. A quick read with important information."

Alan Partin, MD
David Hall McConnell Professor and Chair
Urologist-in-Chief, Department of Urology, Oncology
Johns Hopkins Medical Institutions
Baltimore, MD

Patients' Guide to
Prostate Cancer

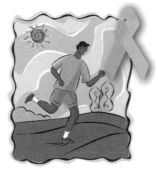

Arthur L. Burnett, MD, MBA, FACS

Patrick C. Walsh Professor of Urology, Cellular and Molecular Medicine
The James Buchanan Brady Urological Institute
The Johns Hopkins Hospital
Baltimore, MD

SERIES EDITORS

Lillie D. Shockney, RN, BS, MAS

University Distinguished Service Associate Professor of Breast Cancer;
Administrative Director of Breast Cancer; Associate Professor, Department of Surgery; Associate
Professor, Department of Obstetrics and Gynecology, Johns Hopkins School of Medicine; Associate
Professor, Johns Hopkins School of Nursing
Baltimore, MD

Gary R. Shapiro, MD

Chairman, Department of Oncology
Johns Hopkins Bayview Medical Center
Director, Johns Hopkins Geriatric Oncology Program
The Sidney Kimmel Comprehensive Cancer Center at Johns Hopkins
Baltimore, MD

JONES AND BARTLETT PUBLISHERS
Sudbury, Massachusetts
BOSTON   TORONTO   LONDON   SINGAPORE

World Headquarters

Jones and Bartlett Publishers
40 Tall Pine Drive
Sudbury, MA 01776
978-443-5000
info@jbpub.com
www.jbpub.com

Jones and Bartlett Publishers
Canada
6339 Ormindale Way
Mississauga, Ontario L5V 1J2
Canada

Jones and Bartlett Publishers
International
Barb House, Barb Mews
London W6 7PA
United Kingdom

Jones and Bartlett's books and products are available through most bookstores and online booksellers. To contact Jones and Bartlett Publishers directly, call 800-832-0034, fax 978-443-8000, or visit our website, www.jbpub.com.

Substantial discounts on bulk quantities of Jones and Bartlett's publications are available to corporations, professional associations, and other qualified organizations. For details and specific discount information, contact the special sales department at Jones and Bartlett via the above contact information or send an email to specialsales@jbpub.com.

The authors, editor, and publisher have made every effort to provide accurate information. However, they are not responsible for errors, omissions, or for any outcomes related to the use of the contents of this book and take no responsibility for the use of the products and procedures described. Treatments and side effects described in this book may not be applicable to all people; likewise, some people may require a dose or experience a side effect that is not described herein. Drugs and medical devices are discussed that may have limited availability controlled by the Food and Drug Administration (FDA) for use only in a research study or clinical trial. Research, clinical practice, and government regulations often change the accepted standard in this field. When consideration is being given to use of any drug in the clinical setting, the healthcare provider or reader is responsible for determining FDA status of the drug, reading the package insert, and reviewing prescribing information for the most up-to-date recommendations on dose, precautions, and contraindications, and determining the appropriate usage for the product. This is especially important in the case of drugs that are new or seldom used.

Production Credits
Executive Publisher: Christopher Davis
Editorial Assistant: Sara Cameron
Production Director: Amy Rose
Production Editor: Dan Stone
Senior Marketing Manager: Barb Bartoszek
V.P., Manufacturing and Inventory Control: Therese Connell
Composition: Auburn Associates, Inc.
Printing and Binding: Malloy, Inc.
Cover Printing: Malloy, Inc.
Cover Design: Kristin E. Parker
Cover Image: © Image Zoo/age fotostock

Library of Congress Cataloging-in-Publication Data

Burnett, Arthur.
   The Johns Hopkins patients' guide to prostate cancer / Arthur Burnett.
      p. cm.—(The Johns Hopkins patients' guide series)
   Includes index.
   ISBN-13: 978-0-7637-7459-2
   ISBN-10: 0-7637-7459-6
   1. Prostate—Cancer—Popular works. I. Title.
   RC280.P7B87 2010
   616.99'463—dc22

                                                          2009022823

6048

Printed in the United States of America
14 13 12 11 10   10 9 8 7 6 5 4 3 2 1

This book is dedicated foremost to my parents
whose love, support and display of character
prepared me; and also to all my mentors whose
wise counsel and examples of excellence
further influenced my life's contributions.

Table of Contents

Preface

Prostate cancer is a formidable foe, but it need not defeat us. No doubt it is a daunting disease developing as a clinical threat to life in as many as 1 in 6 men in the United States. Added to this major statistic (one of many for this disease) is the dilemma associated with various controversies frequently advertised about it—from accepting the utility of available diagnostic tests to defining the risk-benefit optimum for assorted treatments. All of this does create a certain "solemnness," if not confusion, surrounding the disease for many, and certainly for patients and their families who are confronted with it.

Taking action to understand prostate cancer, and gaining knowledge about it to make informed management decisions, is a proper course of action to respond to the challenge of the disease. This book is meant to provide insight and guidance in this regard. Hopefully, its content will be empowering to you—enough to take on the enemy and defeat it. I salute you for being proactive in seeking the best management possible and partnering with your trusted medical professional consultant to succeed.

Arthur L. Burnett, MD, MBA, FACS

Introduction

How to Use This Book to Your Benefit

You will receive a great deal of information from your healthcare team. You will also probably seek out some information on the Internet or in bookstores. No doubt friends and family members, meaning well, will offer you advice on what to do and when to do it, and will try to steer you in certain directions. Relax. Yes, you have heard words you wish you had never heard said about you, that you have prostate cancer. Despite this shocking phrase, you have time to make good decisions and to empower yourself with accurate information so that you can participate in the decision making about your care and treatment.

This book is designed to be a how-to guide that will take you through the maze of treatment options and sometimes complicated schedules, and will help you put together a plan of action so that you become a prostate cancer survivor.

The majority of men diagnosed today will be survivors of this disease. Your goal is to join that majority.

This book is broken down into chapters and includes an index as well as credible resources listed for your further review and education. By empowering yourself with understandable information, we hope you will be comfortable participating in the decision making about your treatment.

You don't need to rush into treatment immediately. You have time on your side to plan things well and confidently. Let's begin now with understanding what has happened and what the steps are to get you well again.

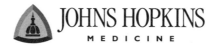
JOHNS HOPKINS
M E D I C I N E

First Steps— I've Been Diagnosed with Prostate Cancer

A diagnosis of prostate cancer was made. At the time of your routine annual physical examination, suspicion was raised either because of an elevation in your serum prostate-specific antigen (PSA) level or an abnormality of the prostate noted by digital rectal examination. No doubt, this is an emotional shock. At the same time, the diagnosis might not seem all that surprising based on population studies that suggest that the current risk of diagnosis of prostate cancer approximates 1 in 6 men in the United States. Prostate cancer is the most commonly diagnosed malignancy among men in the United States, with approximately 200,000 diagnoses a year and approximately 30,000 deaths annually. The numbers are all the more daunting for black men, who have a 40% higher risk of the disease and twice the rate of death from it. According to current statistics, approximately 1 in 38 men will die from prostate cancer. On a positive note, the mortality rate associated with this disease has declined over the past decade. The reduced mortality is associated with various factors, including screening efforts leading to earlier detection and advances in life-saving therapeutic approaches.

Multiple controversies surround the diagnosis of prostate cancer. With better detection, the prevalence of prostate cancer has risen, though in up to 50 percent of men, it may not be life threatening and require active treatment. Thus, a logical question is whether all prostate cancer is deadly? Another is whether active treatment may carry more hazards, such as side effects that hamper quality of life, than the threat of this disease? Today, treatment decisions must take into account a careful understanding of the risk profile of the diagnosis in each man as well as issues regarding his overall health status and life expectancy. A variety of treatments exist, but choice of intervention—from surgery to active surveillance—will differ among patients. Certainly, you may have heard about many of these controversies, which likely adds to your anxiety and fear. The stress may be further heightened because of the idea today that patients should assume a more active role in the decision-making process for managing their disease.

HOW TO SELECT YOUR ONCOLOGY TEAM AND MEDICAL CENTER

It is well documented that the best outcomes associated with prostate cancer management are related to the qualifications of your treating physicians and medical center. It makes sense to consider a medical center for your management that has a high level commitment to prostate cancer management and that provides a diversity of personnel and resources dedicated to patients with prostate cancer. The facility may be a referral center separate from where your prostate cancer diagnosis was made under the care of your original urologist. This facility may include a urologic surgeon with expertise in prostate cancer, radiation oncologist, medical oncologist, prostate pathologist, prostate imaging radiologist, genetics counselors, oncology nurses, and a psychosocial support staff for patients diagnosed with prostate cancer. There should be interaction between all these specialists in the form of interdisciplinary conferences and tumor boards, during which the latest developments in management of both common and complicated cases are discussed. Such a center offers the very latest and best treatments that have been established through rigorous studies as well as the option to be involved in active clinical trials forecasting new therapies.

LEARNING ABOUT YOUR DISEASE BEFORE THE FIRST VISIT

It is important to know that prostate cancer does not always carry the death sentence that it once did. Because of the routine use of PSA testing, prostate cancer is often found very early, and it is estimated that many men may have as much as a 10-year advance notice of the disease. To appreciate this concept further, consider that today 1 in 20 men presenting with prostate cancer diagnoses have distant metastases, compared with the rate of 1 in 3 men who presented with the disease in 1982. This "lead time effect" enables early action. Of course, it also raises challenges for considering whether the diagnosis always merits active treatment that may carry risks (see previous discussion). Nonetheless, having an early start by knowing you have the diagnosis may be the best position to be in so that you and your doctors can plan for the very best outcome.

GATHERING RECORDS: BIOPSY, LABS, RADIOLOGY REPORTS

In preparing for another consultation, it is important to collect your medical records and other pertinent information to bring with you for your consultation. These records should specifically assist in the evaluation of your prostate cancer risk profile. However, other records may also be helpful for the evaluation of your overall health status that may affect the best recommendation. Regarding prostate health records, serial PSA testing over many years may have been done, and results showing the trend in these measurements could be very helpful. The prostate biopsy report detailing specifics about the biopsy findings should be copied and brought. Specific information from the biopsy includes the number of biopsy cores obtained, the locations of biopsy cores containing cancer within the prostate, the percentage of cancer within each biopsy core, and the determination of Gleason score (a grading system that defines the appearance of the cancerous tissue).

For many centers, the actual biopsy slides containing your tissue are requested for first-hand review by pathologists at the medical center to render an independent evaluation of your prostate cancer. Sending these slides in advance for pathologic review or having them on hand with you during the initial consultation can be very helpful to move along the pathologic review process. Additionally, reports of any imaging studies such as bone scan, CAT scan, or MRI may be shown. In the past, these additional imaging studies were frequently ordered, but today they are not commonly done in men with an early diagnosis and evidence of only localized disease. Medical records from your previous urologic consultations can also be very helpful, particularly to review any initial treatments that you may have received. Knowing what has already been done for your prostate cancer may affect further decisions regarding management. Brief summaries of your overall medical conditions are also useful. Your doctors will want to take into account your other health problems so they can recommend the best treatment for your prostate cancer. As stated earlier, the natural history of prostate cancer can be long and drawn out. For many men, their other medical conditions will have a greater effect on their health and longevity than will their prostate cancer diagnosis. In these men, less urgent or aggressive prostate cancer management may be the most appropriate course. It is important to avoid implementing major interventions when they may be unnecessary.

CANCER STAGING

Clinical staging is an important component of the initial evaluation. Clinical stage refers to the extent of the disease and as such influences decision making because it indicates how far the disease has progressed and how likely a treatment may be able to control it. Other components of the initial evaluation include two readily available clinical diagnostic variables: the PSA level and the Gleason score from the prostate biopsy. Often, these variables are combined to give the probability of the progression of disease. Tools used for this purpose include predictive, validated nomograms. Such nomograms provide information regarding the likelihood that the disease is confined to the prostate gland, spread locally beyond the prostate gland, or spread distantly into lymph node tissue or elsewhere in the body. Many patients have a heightened appreciation of their prostate cancer risk profile by accessing nomograms and then entering in their own clinical variables to get a sense of the "big picture."

The most common form of prostate cancer is adenocarcinoma (greater than 95%). This type of prostate cancer is a malignant transformation of the structure of glands and the cells that make up these glands into a random and disorganized architecture. Prostate cancer tissue can be evaluated under the microscope to identify this transformation. The pathologist's microscopic evaluation of the prostate cancer tissue also determines the aggressiveness level, referred to as the Gleason score. The Gleason score represents the sum of two numbers rating the two most common patterns of abnormal glandular architecture based on a graded scale of 1 to 5, with 1 indicating low-grade cancer and 5 indicating high-grade cancer. The first number corresponds with the predominant pattern and the second number relating to the second most common pattern observed in examining the prostate tissue for an individual patient. For example, a Gleason score of $4 + 3 = 7$ indicates a predominant pattern of mostly abnormal glands that are not quite the highest grade with a secondary pattern that is somewhat less. In cases where the glands are abnormal but still fairly uniform in appearance, the same number may be repeated. Tumor aggressiveness increases with the score (e.g., 4 + 4 is more aggressive than 3 + 4).

When doctors refer to cancer staging they are talking about the extent to which the cancer has spread. Both "clinical staging" and "pathological staging" are frequently used, but it is important to recognize the difference between them. Clinical staging refers to the determination of the extent of disease based on clinical findings prior to any sort of treatment. This primarily involves the findings from the digital rectal examination. Digital rectal examination assesses whether the tumor is palpable and the extent to which this seems to involve the prostate. Because the prostate is a bilobar structure, the examiner can comment on whether the tumor is minimally or extensively palpable, and if it involves one or both sides of the prostate. This palpation involves only the zone of the prostate that borders on the rectal wall, and this side of the prostate is called the peripheral zone. Prostate cancer may also arise in areas of the prostate that are not accessible to the examiner's finger. This limitation may account for the difference that may occur between clinical and pathological staging. When they are indicated, imaging studies may provide further information to determine the extent of disease. Bone scan, pelvic CAT scan or MRI may increase the original clinical stage that was determined only by digital rectal examination.

Pathological staging, on the other hand, indicates the extent of cancer that is found in the surgically removed tissue specimens. Pathological staging requires surgery so the pathologist can evaluate the removed prostate to directly assess the extent of cancer spread. Pelvic lymph nodes are also regularly removed during surgery and then assessed for cancer spread.

A review of the various ways that PSA testing aids the clinical evaluation of prostate cancer is helpful. The PSA level itself is helpful, and it is quite readily understood that the higher the number the greater the extent of disease and worse prognosis. But, there are exceptions. Tumors that are poorly differentiated (extremely different from normal biological tissue) may not produce significant amounts of PSA such that the measurement in blood may seem surprisingly low. On the other hand, there are cases in which a more elevated PSA measurement can occur with a large amount of cancerous tissue present within the prostate in locations that may not easily be appreciated on the digital rectal examination, such as the anterior zone (opposite to the peripheral zone).

A complicating issue is that the PSA test is not cancer specific. The test is only prostate specific, and elevations may arise from benign diseases of the prostate such as benign prostatic enlargement and prostatitis. Other forms of PSA measurement have been developed in an attempt to correct for elevations associated with benign conditions of the prostate. These include PSA density, free PSA, and PSA velocity. These are briefly explained as follows. PSA density is a measurement of the PSA level divided by estimation of prostate volume determined by transrectal ultrasonography and simply implies that the PSA value is adjusted for prostate size. A PSA density of less than 0.1 generally implies a low risk situation for prostate cancer. Free PSA refers to a molecular form of PSA that is not bound to a circulating protein in the blood called alpha$_1$-antichymotrypsin. The free PSA measurement is generally higher in men with benign disease, and a measurement of less than 15% suggests clinically significant or more aggressive disease. PSA velocity refers to the change in PSA over time. The greater the rate of PSA increases over time, the greater the threat of a clinically adverse form of prostate cancer. A PSA change of greater than 2 ng/ml in the year before diagnosis means an increased risk of death from prostate cancer.

CHAPTER 2

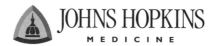

My Team—
MEETING YOUR
TREATMENT TEAM

PLAYERS

Many different individuals comprise your professional team. These include the prostate cancer urologic surgeon, radiation oncologist, medical oncologist, pathologist, radiologist, nurses, social worker, and others. The following best describes the roles of these individuals:

Prostate Cancer Urologic Surgeon. This is a physician with surgical expertise in performing radical prostatectomy, the removal of the prostate, appropriate surrounding tissue, and pelvic lymph nodes. Oftentimes, this is the first doctor you will see for the diagnosis and initial management of your disease. This specialist may also perform other types of pelvic surgery for the treatment of prostate cancer that do not involve prostate removal (see discussion in Chapter 3).

Radiation oncologist. This specialist evaluates the role of radiation therapy and implements this therapy if a decision is made that the tumor is best treated by irradiation.

Medical oncologist. This specialist becomes involved once treatments that require complicated medicine regimens such as chemotherapy, hormonal therapy, and any possibly novel combination therapies are considered. This doctor may not necessarily be the initial physician carrying out your evaluation. The medical oncologist's role is more significant for patients with advanced prostate cancer.

Pathologist. This is a specialist in the evaluation of the tissue specimens that are retrieved, by biopsy or surgery, during your evaluation and management. The pathologist examines the tissue specimens under the microscope to facilitate an accurate assessment of the tumor aggressiveness and extent.

Radiologist. This specialist is involved in studying and describing findings demonstrated by imaging studies (like x-rays, bone scans, CAT scans, and MRI scans) used in the evaluation and staging of prostate cancer.

Nurses. Nurses are professionals providing important roles in the overall care of prostate cancer patients. They also serve as counselors and educators for both patients and families.

Social Worker. This team player is involved in support issues surrounding the management of prostate cancer. The social worker may also be involved in addressing financial concerns that arise surrounding clinical management.

Survivor volunteer. This individual may play a very important role for any patient receiving a diagnosis of prostate cancer, considering management options, and proceeding through clinical management. A patient "who has been there before" offers tremendous emotional support and complements the service the professional staff provides.

MAKING YOUR INITIAL APPOINTMENT

Having been given the diagnosis of prostate cancer, you may feel you want to be seen at a major medical center specializing in the management of prostate cancer. It is very appropriate to do so. It makes sense that a high-volume center with many experienced clinicians may be able to bring you the best management for your disease. The medical literature also supports this assumption. You may get a sense that a medical facility is highly reputable for its management of prostate cancer based on published ratings of hospital performances. You may also gather more information using Internet Web sites that describe clinical services available at various medical centers.

Identify a prostate cancer urologic surgeon who has been well trained and specializes in prostate cancer management. The surgeon should be credentialed and Board Certified as a urologist. This surgeon should also have demonstrated additional ability and focus in prostate cancer management. The specialist should be an experienced, highly skilled surgeon who can report on the number of prostate cancer surgeries he/she does on a monthly and yearly basis and the total number of surgeries performed during the course of his/her career. As a rule of thumb, an experienced surgeon should actively perform at least 50 surgeries annually and have accomplished more than 500 surgeries in total. Do not be afraid to ask your surgeon for this information.

Question further to learn about that surgeon's results, what are often refered to as "surgical outcomes." These outcomes include the success in controlling the cancer, based on the pathology results and clinical follow-up. Outcomes related to recovery of sexual function and urinary control are especially important. When you talk to your surgeon be direct and persistent when asking about his/her outcomes. If the surgeon is truly committed to you, he/she should be forthright in explaining all these issues and put you at ease in understanding their relevance. Any dedicated prostate cancer surgeon readily has this information available for discussion.

When you make your appointment, it is important to ask the scheduler what you should do to facilitate your evaluation. Ask if you need to provide your doctor with your medical records, pathology slides, or scans. Many consultants prefer that you send all of your information before the appointment, but the scheduler may tell you that your doctor prefers you to bring it with you. The surgeon may briefly review the pathology slides and then submit them to the pathology department for an official review and report. Some facilities have taken advantage of electronic information to facilitate your evaluation. Your scheduler may inform you that an online electronic medical intake form can be completed and then entered into the medical records system prior to your arrival, thus facilitating your evaluation as well. Taking the time to do this yourself allows you to complete your medical record thoroughly and accurately. It may also allow you to be more relaxed when you go to the medical center. Certainly, you will be very anxious and distracted at times during this consultation, and any "homework" done in advance will be advantageous for you and all involved.

A brief remark should be made about your intent in pursuing a consultation. You owe it to yourself to be thoroughly informed regarding your diagnosis and management options. Your primary medical facility should be helpful in this regard. Upon your request, your initially treating physician's office should facilitate your access to medical records as well as your pathology slides. You are entitled to your medical records as well as your pathology slides; these items are your property. If office workers are reluctant to release your records, pathology slides, or other information, inform them that they will be returned after your consultation. Be persistent, and, if you struggle in any way, you may ask the medical center providing your consultation for help.

QUESTIONS TO ASK DURING YOUR CONSULTATIVE VISIT

In preparation for your visit, you may have a number of questions to assist in your own understanding of your diagnosis and consideration of options for management. To help you get started, here are some questions that should definitely be considered in your discussion with your urologic surgeon or radiation therapist consultant:

1. How quickly do I need to be treated?

2. Is my cancer at an early or late stage of progression?

3. Do I have high risk features associated with my cancer presentation to indicate that I might die from it?

4. What clinical factors are considered to determine how I should proceed?

5. How effective are different treatments in hopes of curing my prostate cancer?

6. Is there anything I can do right now to help reduce the risk of progression of my cancer?

7. What are the risks associated with different treatments?

8. Will my risk profile change after your assessment, including the review of my biopsy slides by the pathologist?

9. What changes in my sexual, urinary, or bowel function may occur following different treatments?

10. What sort of recovery timetable can I expect following surgery before resuming physical exercise or work?

11. What life and work adjustments do I need to make while going through radiation treatments?

12. Will I require special health care assistance in any way during my recuperation following surgery?

13. Will I require additional radiation or hormonal therapy after surgery?

14. Can you determine if I am cured right after the surgery based on surgical observations?

15. Am I a candidate for nerve-sparing surgery, and how likely is this to prevent erectile dysfunction (impotence)?

16. What are the rates and timetable for recovery of physical activities, erectile function, and urinary control after surgery?

17. If I have impairments in erectile or urinary function before surgery or radiation, how will these functions be affected afterward? Better or worse?

18. Are there specialized medications, exercises, or other maneuvers that should be applied soon after treatment or even before treatment to facilitate recovery of erectile function or urinary control?

19. Besides affecting erection, will surgery or radiation affect other aspects of sexual function such as sexual drive, orgasmic function, or even penile dimensions?

20. How do my current health conditions influence outcomes from surgery?

21. Are there clinical trials that I should consider participating in besides standard treatment options for my prostate cancer presentation?

22. What are the advantages and disadvantages of different surgical approaches used to treat prostate cancer?

23. What are the advantages and disadvantages of different radiation therapy approaches used to treat prostate cancer?

24. If I have more questions before my treatment begins, can I contact someone to answer my questions?

25. Will you see me again to review plans for surgery before my surgery day?

WHAT TESTS NEED TO BE DONE

During your initial consultation visit, the consultant may consider doing additional tests to help with the evaluation before making recommendations. A repeat digital rectal examination is often done because the surgeon or radiation therapist may wish to confirm the clinical staging, particularly if there was an earlier observation of palpable cancer on digital rectal examination. The reevaluation may assist the consultant in understanding firsthand the extent of cancer that may affect his/her therapeutic plan. This procedure is very useful for the surgeon whose assessment of the extent of cancer may influence decisions regarding nerve-sparing (preservation of erection-producing nerves surrounding the prostate). A repeat PSA test may be done, although sometimes this is not necessary. It should be recognized that a recent biopsy of the prostate causes PSA tests to be inaccurate. Any PSA value obtained within a month following biopsy should simply be disregarded.

As discussed previously, a repeat pathology review is regularly performed. This procedure offers a true "second opinion" regarding the pathological interpretation of your biopsy slides. The question often arises as to whether a repeat prostate biopsy would be useful. The question is particularly pertinent if your original biopsy showed only minimal findings of prostate cancer, either in terms of minimal extent or low grade of disease. Patients having less than the standard 12-core prostate biopsy may be in this dilemma if pathology results are determined to be less than informative. In this case, a repeat prostate biopsy may be necessary to provide adequate sampling of the prostate that would give a much better indication of the real threat of the disease.

The role of imaging studies has changed dramatically in the past 15 to 20 years because prostate cancer in the United States is now diagnosed at such an early stage. The widespread use of serum PSA testing has resulted in many men receiving an early prostate diagnosis that it is unlikely to have spread throughout the body. Frequently, the standard clinical variables of PSA test, clinical stage, and Gleason score indicate that the cancer is unlikely to have spread. In such situations, additional imaging tests are probably unnecessary since their yield for showing disease spread in the body is very low. Your consultant may discuss this issue with you, and if there are concerns, imaging tests can certainly be ordered. The standard imaging tests are CAT scan of the abdomen and pelvis, as well as a bone scan. Pelvic MRI study is also frequently obtained for clinical staging, and may be most relevant for many radiation therapy recommendations.

Your surgeon may want you to see your primary care provider for a preoperative examination and "medical clearance" to proceed with treatment. Standard preoperative tests include blood work, chest x-ray, and electrocardiogram. The tests are done to ensure that there are no acute health conditions requiring attention prior to undergoing surgery or radiation.

CHAPTER 3

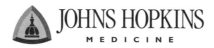

TAKING ACTION— COMPREHENSIVE TREATMENT CONSIDERATIONS

Upon completion of your diagnostic evaluation, recommendations will be made regarding the optimal type of treatment you may receive. Importantly, the distinction between localized and metastatic prostate cancer will immediately dictate treatment considerations. Localized prostate cancer means that there is no extension to the seminal vesicles, regional lymph nodes, or in areas beyond the pelvic region. A patient diagnosed with localized disease is a candidate for one of three forms of therapy: expectant management, surgery, or radiation therapy. A patient diagnosed with metastatic disease (beyond the pelvic region) is a candidate for hormonal therapy or chemotherapy. Localized treatment is for prostate cancer that is of earlier clinical stage and has not spread throughout the body, whereas nonlocalized treatments are required for disease that has spread. Treatment considerations should also include knowledge of the advantages and disadvantages of different treatments, specific goals of treatment for each patient, and patient preferences regarding choice of treatment. An informed patient can contribute to the decision-making process for treatment. A review of treatment options follows.

EXPECTANT MANAGEMENT

As discussed previously, many men will carry a diagnosis of prostate cancer that may not necessarily threaten their life spans. Such men may be considered candidates for expectant management, which also is referred to as active surveillance. The strategy is generally applied to patients who have a life expectancy of less than 10 years and for healthy men 65 years of age or older whose diagnostic work-up suggests low-volume, low-grade prostate cancer. This determination requires the assessment of clinical stage along with PSA test results and findings from your prostate biopsy. Generally, well-accepted criteria include no palpable disease on digital rectal examination, the PSA density (the PSA level divided by the prostate sonographic volume) is below 0.15, the "free" PSA level is above 15%, and there should be less than 3 biopsy cores showing a tumor with a Gleason score below 7 and no core showing more than 50% involvement.

As suggested by the terminology, expectant management means that a patient has his prostate cancer monitored for signs of progression by standardized clinical evaluations done on a set schedule. A recommended approach is to undergo digital rectal examinations and PSA testing twice a year, and prostate biopsies annually. If these test findings show that the prostate cancer has advancement beyond "low threat" disease, active treatment may be required. Presumably, moving forward to active treatment at this time should still cure the prostate cancer. Approximately 25% of men managed expectantly will advance beyond "low threat" prostate cancer. This percentage is substantial and suggests that such conservative management may not be ideal for patients younger than 65 years of age. Unlike older men with decreased life expectancy, younger men may miss the opportunity for cure if they are not treated aggressively.

Concern about the best way to manage the man whose prostate cancer has progressed during expectant management is certainly justified. Would an aggressive approach suddenly be worth implementing in this instance? A more conservative approach could still be applied when disease progression is identified, particularly for a man 65 years of age or older with possible adverse health conditions and relatively decreased life expectancy. These conservative options include transurethral resection of the prostate (using an instrument inserted through the penis to scrape out cancerous tissue interfering with urination), radiation therapy, and hormonal therapy. These interventions are not meant to be curative and are initiated to control the disease so that it is unlikely to cause this man's death.

SURGERY

In a man with localized disease that truly threatens his life, surgery for removal of the prostate has been a mainstay of treatment. The intent of this intervention is to remove the entire prostate and seminal vesicles along with surrounding tissue so that all disease is eradicated. The surgical management may also involve removal of pelvic lymph nodes, situated on both sides (bilaterally) of the prostate, where prostate cancer may spread. The standard terminology used for this procedure is radical prostatectomy with bilateral pelvic lymph node dissection. The role of this surgical procedure is meant to be aggressive in hopes that a curative outcome is met. Indeed, when the cancer is truly confined to the prostate, the perceived advantage of radical prostatectomy results from the total removal of the prostate gland by the surgery.

Today, several surgical options are commonly used for removing the prostate gland. These include open retropubic and perineal approaches as well as laparoscopic approaches with or without robotic assistance (involving multiple stab-like incisions for passage of instruments).

For a man considering radical prostatectomy, the range of surgical approaches may seem bewildering. How is one to know which surgical approach is the best? The answer is actually fairly straightforward. All approaches can be applied successfully with minimal surgical risk, with the caveat that, besides the characteristics of the cancer itself, surgical expertise is the most important feature in determining outcome. That is to say, when a highly skilled surgeon performs the surgery, any approach will likely achieve comparable outcomes; both with regard to cancer control and recovery of functional abilities, including urinary and sexual functions (see Chapter 4).

Functional recovery following radical prostatectomy remains an everlasting concern. This concern applies to any of the surgical approaches used to perform a radical prostatectomy. The prostate gland is situated in a precarious place in the body, adjacent to the urinary sphincter for urinary control (urinary continence), the cavernous nerves coursing in the pelvis to the penis responsible for penile erection, and the rectum and anal sphincter with importance for bowel function. Understandably, surgery to remove the prostate stands the risk that one or more of these bodily functions may be affected. The approach to surgery is meant to preserve pelvic structures and restore these structures to the best extent possible such that functional losses do not occur. Innovations such as "nerve-sparing" refinements of radical prostatectomy have had major importance in the application of surgery, particularly with relevance to preserving a man's potency. Other refinements such as identification and surgical control of pelvic blood vessels and proper dissection (anatomical separation) of the urinary sphincter have also led to improvements in the surgery and better outcomes.

Currently, statistics show that radical prostatectomy allows for the best cancer control and functional outcomes. Less than 2% of patients with true early stage disease (pathological findings that the cancer is confined to the prostate gland) should ever have positive margins (pathological evidence that cancer exists at any of the surgical specimen boundaries). With the proper application of surgical refinements, clinically significant urinary incontinence (loss of urinary control) should occur in only about 3% of men and clinically significant erectile dysfunction (impotence) should occur in approximately 30% of men. These statistics are consistent with outcomes reported from major medical centers specializing in prostate cancer management. Higher complication rates have been reported, which does "cloud the picture" regarding expectations following surgery. Many factors may influence these reported high rates, including inconsistent definitions of functional conditions and imperfect assessments of functional recovery, although proper knowledge and execution of the surgery remain dominant features affecting the best outcomes. The wise advice here is that you should indeed seek out the most qualified surgeon possible who by any surgical approach will expectedly produce the very best possible results for you.

RADIATION THERAPY

Radiation therapy represents another option to treat localized prostate cancer. Two main forms of radiation therapy are external beam radiotherapy and interstitial seed (brachytherapy) radiotherapy. External beam radiation is delivered from a source outside of the body, and involves multiple treatment sessions. It uses conformal techniques that deliver the radiation waves more focally and reduce the likelihood of radiation spread to structures beyond the prostate gland. Brachytherapy involves the surgical placement of radiated seeds (radioactive iodine-125 or palladium-102 seeds) into the prostate. Both external beam and brachytherapy techniques rely upon imaging procedures to ensure that the radiation is delivered as accurately as possible.

Because radiation therapy is noninvasive or minimally invasive in its approach, it is perceived to be more advantageous than surgery. By being less intrusive to the body, it is believed that radiation is less traumatic to structures of the body. Some side effects of treatment may also be potentially minimized such as severe urinary incontinence associated with urinary sphincter damage. Radiation therapy may also offer a strategic approach for managing prostate cancer that is locally spread beyond the prostate but is not amenable to surgical management. In such cases, the prostate cancer may have spread in such a way that complete removal of the cancer is not possible without significant damage to local structures surrounding the prostate. Radiation therapy then may help control the disease in this more locally advanced disease state. Despite these advantages, radiation therapy, like surgery, carries the potential for complication risks (see Chapter 4). Side effects are related to radiation wave scatter to structures surrounding the prostate that have to do with other bodily functions such as urinary, bowel, and sexual functions. As with surgery, refinements in radiation for prostate cancer have reduced complication rates. Specialized techniques may be available at major medical centers with facilities and experience that limit doses of radiation to surrounding structures.

HORMONAL THERAPY

Hormonal therapy, also known as androgen deprivation therapy, is an option for managing prostate cancer that is too advanced for surgery or radiation therapy. Because prostate cancer cells thrive on the male hormone testosterone, strategies that withdraw testosterone cause prostate cancer cells to grow and spread less rapidly. This intervention offers a way to manage prostate cancer cells that have metastasized to areas in the body beyond the pelvic region; including, lymph node tissue, bones, and other vital organs.

There are two major ways of providing hormonal therapy. One approach is orchiectomy. This is a surgical procedure to remove the testicles from the scrotum. The testicles are the main source of testosterone in the body. Another approach uses medications that suppress testosterone production or its action throughout the body. This medication may be delivered in various forms ranging from oral medications to injections.

Controversy surrounds the timing for using hormonal therapy. Clearly, for the man with advanced prostate cancer that is symptomatic, including bone pain, weight loss changes, or a general sense of ill-being, hormonal therapy may be started to treat these symptoms. However, for the man who is not symptomatic, recommendations have ranged from early hormonal therapy to delay progression of disease, to starting treatment only when symptoms develop or there are concerns about rapid disease progression. Experts who support delayed hormonal therapy acknowledge that limited evidence supports any significant improvement in survival rate based on early hormonal treatment. Furthermore, symptoms can occur in men using hormonal therapy, which must be balanced against goals of the treatment. Symptoms include hot flashes, fatigue, decreased erectile ability, decreased sexual libido, breast tenderness, loss of bone mass, loss of muscle mass, decreased mental acuity, and risk for development of metabolic disorders such as diabetes.

Although hormonal therapy is generally associated with the management of metastatic prostate cancer, it may also have a role when radiation therapy is used to treat locally advanced prostate cancer. Clinical studies have shown that when hormonal treatment is given prior to radiation therapy, outcomes for disease control are better than when radiation is given alone. Hormonal therapy may create this advantage by reducing tumor size or otherwise sensitizing tumor cells to subsequent radiation administration.

CHEMOTHERAPY

Chemotherapy, medications administered for cancer cells that have spread within the body, also serves an important purpose in managing advanced prostate cancer. Hormonal therapy has its limitations because it only slows the progression of prostate cancer cells and does not effectively rid the body of these cells. With this knowledge, investigators have been conscientious in exploring chemotherapeutic possibilities for advanced prostate cancer. However, advances have been slow because prostate cancer cells have been shown to be quite resistant to chemotherapy (chemoresistant). The recent development of the drug Taxotere is a breakthrough for the chemotherapeutic management of prostate cancer. This drug has been used with some success in improving survival in some men. Side effects from this medication include fatigue, weight loss, and bowel disturbances. Other chemotherapeutic drugs have been explored with seemingly less effectiveness. These also may produce side effects. Nevertheless, many of these side effects can be overcome with treatments like antinausea medicines. As studies continue to improve our understanding about how prostate cancer cells progress and spread, there is hope for the development of better chemotherapeutic agents that target the biological conditions of this disease.

OTHER TREATMENTS

Conventional treatment options for clinically localized prostate cancer should be explored first because of their known treatment efficacies. However, recent proposals have been made for the possible application of two minimally invasive forms of therapy for this disease. One option is cryotherapy, which involves freezing procedures to destroy prostate tissue. The other is high-intensity focused ultrasonography, which involves the application of a heated beam of focused ultrasound waves guided to the prostate by an ultrasound probe that is placed into the rectum. This approach also leads to prostate tissue destruction. Conceptually, both offer alternatives with the assumption that the cancer will be sufficiently treated and complication risks minimized. However, sufficient data to substantiate claims for either position is not yet available.

Additional thought has been given to whether adjuvant systemic therapy (chemotherapy or hormonal therapy) could be applied immediately after surgery or radiation for localized prostate cancer. The notion is that such additional therapy may afford patients better opportunities for disease control if they are considered to be at high risk for recurrence. However, definitive answers in this regard are also lacking.

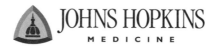

CHAPTER 4

JOHNS HOPKINS
MEDICINE

BE PREPARED—
THE SIDE EFFECTS OF TREATMENT

Once you have been diagnosed with prostate cancer, you should be prepared to contemplate all aspects regarding management options. It is important to be informed not just about the possible roles of different treatment options and their effectiveness but also about their possible side effects. A balanced and complete understanding of all facets of management regarding your prostate cancer diagnosis including the risks of various treatments is recommended. Being informed in such a way may influence your final decisions regarding management.

A discussion of management complications deserves particular attention for prostate cancer, no less than for any other cancer diagnosis. In particular, the concern has to do with treatments for localized prostate cancer (disease confined to the prostate or its immediate surrounding area).

The prostate is precariously positioned in the deep pelvis adjacent to pelvic structures that are involved in urination, defecation, and sexual functions. Therefore, treatments for localized prostate cancer risk affecting these functions.

The history of treatments for prostate cancer well illustrates the concern for these functional losses. In men who underwent surgery or radiation in the past, substantial numbers incurred urinary incontinence that required the use of pads or diapers after treatment. It was also common for them to lose the ability to achieve reliable erections for sexual activity. Such risks likely accounted for many men shunning treatments and others forgoing clinical evaluations for a possible prostate cancer diagnosis. The enduring consequences of advanced disease (e.g., body weakness, weight loss, and other effects of cancer spread in the body) were preferred to experiencing any alteration in one's quality of life.

Fortunately, progress has been made, and these advances have minimized complications so that patients now have a much brighter outlook for retaining normal bodily functions after treatment. Complications have been reduced by improved understanding of the pelvic anatomy, and by advances in doctors' expertise in all forms of prostate cancer treatment. Despite this progress, treatment complications can occur, and it is important to be informed of these when deciding upon and undergoing your prostate cancer treatment. A review of potential complications for prostate cancer follows.

SURGERY

Potential complications of radical prostatectomy have always been at the forefront of concerns of men undergoing localized prostate cancer treatment. The immediate impact of cure resulting from complete removal of the prostate may be accompanied by precipitous and serious surgical side effects. No doubt, at least some extent of temporary erection loss and urinary incontinence occur in all men following the surgery. These major side effects are daunting problems for any man to accept when undergoing this form of treatment.

Complications of surgery can be related to timing—with risks that may occur during the surgery (intraoperative complications) and risks that may occur after the surgery (postoperative complications). It will be helpful to consider these complications in the discussion that follows.

The most common complication occurring during surgery is excessive bleeding. This risk is associated with cutting across blood vessels coursing within the pelvis and around the prostate. Surgery performed in the deep pelvis is very challenging, and a thorough understanding of the anatomical locations of these blood vessels is necessary to perform this surgery with the least possible risk of major surgical bleeding. Presently, this risk is believed to be significantly reduced, and in expert surgical hands there is infrequent need for blood transfusion. The newer approaches of laparoscopic and robotic surgery for radical prostatectomy employ a technique of carbon dioxide gas infusion within the abdomen that creates a pressure effect that may also limit bleeding risk for these approaches.

Other potential intraoperative risks include injury to structures surrounding the prostate such as the rectum or ureters. These risks are fairly uncommon. Predisposing factors are known to influence their occurrences. Anatomical variations, local cancer progression, and prior surgery of the prostate such as a transurethral prostate resection for benign prostate enlargement or multiple biopsies in the past may constitute hazards. If injury to local structures is recognized during surgery, the surgeon should typically be able to carry out an immediate repair. Again, as for intraoperative bleeding, surgical expertise reduces the likelihood of these risks. Finally, the risk of death is always a concern for any surgery involving anesthesia, but this occurrence during radical prostatectomy is thought to be extremely rare (1 in 1000).

After surgery, several complications may develop. Foremost among these are problems with urinary control and sexual function.

Urinary control problems, also known as urinary incontinence, are commonplace following the surgery and have major quality of life implications. The reason urinary incontinence occurs is because the urinary outlet region is changed in the course of performing radical prostatectomy. In men, three zones are normally active to be continent of one's urine. These include the external urinary sphincter (located just beyond the prostate at the pelvic floor), the prostate (located more internally), and the junction of the prostate with the bladder neck (even more internally). As a requirement of surgery, the latter two zones are altered. The surgeon is then required to reconstruct the bladder neck and connect it to the urinary sphincter. A catheter transversing this reconstruction is placed during surgery allowing the area to heal. Once the catheter is removed several days later, almost all men experience at least temporary urinary incontinence. For some men, urinary incontinence may be very brief, and they achieve very good urinary control almost from the moment the catheter is removed. As time goes on with healing and recovery of urinary sphincter strength, a majority of the remaining men recover full urinary control. Commonly, pads or diapers are used during recovery, and their use may continue for a few months in some men. Current rates of recovery of urinary control are approximately 80% of men at 3 months and 97% of men at 12 months after radical prostatectomy.

The success of this recovery may be due to several factors. Simply enough, some men are fortunate to have better urinary sphincter strength than others, and some also may recover their sphincter function faster than others. Many men also are proactive in performing pelvic floor strengthening exercises that may strengthen the external urinary sphincter and speed up the recovery of urinary control. Briefly stated, this is an exercise routine where the patient deliberately stops his urinary stream for 5 to 10 second intervals while he is urinating. It should also be recognized that men who experience urinary abnormalities prior to surgery, whether or not related to an enlarged prostate, may continue to experience such problems afterward. This is particularly of concern for the man with a hyperactive bladder that is associated with sensations of urinary urgency and frequency. A slow urinary stream that occurs following surgery could be associated with abnormal healing of the urinary outlet reconstruction, also known as a bladder neck contracture. This may develop because of scar tissue formation around the reconnected bladder and urethra. Your surgeon should assist you in managing your urinary issues following radical prostatectomy. With proper clinical follow-up, recommendations will be made for pelvic floor strengthening exercises, and any medications that may be required. Additional surgery is sometimes necessary to restore urinary control.

Sexual ability may also be affected by surgery. The major complication is erectile dysfunction (impotence), the loss of the ability to achieve erections for sexual intercourse. Other sexual dysfunctions may also occur as a consequence of surgery. Ejaculation does not occur following surgery once the prostate and seminal vesicles have been removed. However, most men are able to experience satisfying orgasmic sensations despite the ejaculatory loss. Some men may experience changes in their orgasmic function or have painful sensations with orgasm. Changes in the dimensions and structure of the penis (i.e., penile atrophy) may also occur following surgery. Some of these effects are not very well understood, and fortunately for those men experiencing orgasmic pain, this problem will lessen over time.

For erectile dysfunction, trauma of the erection-producing nerves surrounding the prostate during surgery is well understood to affect the erection process. Innovations in preserving the erection-producing nerves have lessened the long-term side effect of erectile dysfunction. However, many men may experience at least some short-term erectile dysfunction. The rate of recovery of penile erections remains a matter of considerable debate in the literature. Reports of erection recovery range between 0% and 90%, allowing for a recovery time as much as two years after surgery. Several factors are known to influence erection recovery. These include patient factors such as age and the level of erectile function before surgery. The local extent of the disease is also important, because this may require the surgical removal of more tissue, which in turn affects the nerves required for erection. The surgeon's ability to perform the operation to preserve the erection-producing nerves (when the circumstances of the cancer presentation are limited enough to allow it) is also critical. The recovery of erections following surgery generally requires natural healing. At this time, there is little convincing evidence that any particular intervention offers a more rapid or complete recovery of natural erectile function. During the recovery process, several interventions are available, and these may be effective in different ways depending upon one's level of erectile function over the course of recovery. Treatment options range from assorted medications (e.g., oral phosphodiesterase type 5 inhibitors such as Viagra®, Cialis® and Levitra®, intraurethral or intracavernosal vasoactive drugs) to various devices (e.g., vacuum erection devices, penile implants) that may be employed under the direction of your urologist.

It is important to recognize additional complications that may occur following radical prostatectomy that are not so well publicized. The development of blood clots in the legs occurs commonly enough, and it may have a potentially very serious risk. Blood clots may form in the lower legs because of changes in blood circulation following radical prostatectomy (as may happen with any sort of pelvic surgery). Some may become dislodged and then circulate to the lungs in the form of a pulmonary embolism. Pulmonary emboli can be fatal, in about 2 in 100 men.

Precautions are taken during surgery to limit the formation of blood clots in the legs. These include the intraoperative and postoperative use of leg stockings that gently compress the lower legs and thereby reduce the opportunity for blood to pool in leg veins. Mechanical compression devices that gently squeeze blood back up the leg and into the body, are also used. Getting up and walking as soon as possible after surgery and dorsiflexion exercises (up and down movements of the feet when reclining in a chair or in bed) pump blood from the legs to the body, and thereby decrease the risk of blood clots forming. In some men who are known to have blood clotting disorders, preventive approaches using blood-thinning medications may be applied according to a well-planned protocol around the time of surgery.

RADIATION THERAPY

External beam radiotherapy and brachytherapy also carry potential complications. Although radiation therapy appeals to many men because it is less invasive than surgery, and generally has few major immediate complications, significant risks may still be encountered.

During the course of radiation therapy, several symptoms may occur that are believed to be generally mild in extent. Fatigue may occur, but, even during the weeks of active treatment, many men are able to tolerate this side effect while carrying on their occupational activities. Urinary symptoms also occur. Most commonly these are described as irritative, causing a man to have a sensation of urinary urgency or urinary frequency. These symptoms may occur in as many as 25% to 30% of men undergoing radiation treatments. While these may be tolerated by the majority of men, some may require medications, at least temporarily, to offset the symptoms. Rectal symptoms may also occur following radiation, and these may range from a sensation to move one's bowels to the experience of multiple daily loose bowel movements.

Complications may occur at some later interval following radiation treatments as well. Both urinary and rectal symptoms may persist in some men even weeks after radiation treatments have been discontinued. Chronic rectal problems may occur in as many as 2 in 100 men, including rectal inflammation, diarrhea, rectal bleeding, and development of an anal stricture. Sexual function may also be impacted adversely as a result of radiation treatments. Erectile dysfunction may occur in up to 60% of patients. As for men undergoing radical prostatectomy, various factors affect the rates of erection recovery following radiation treatments. These include preoperative erectile function status, age, progression of disease locally, and the manner of the radiation treatments. It is noteworthy that the loss of erections with radiation treatments tends to be slow in their onset, which differs with that following radical prostatectomy. In the end, the rates of erectile dysfunction among different treatments may not differ much. Other sexual impairments such as penile deformities and altered orgasmic function have also been reported with radiation treatments.

HORMONAL THERAPY

Hormonal therapy used for advanced prostate cancer also carries the potential for side effects. The most commonly described side effects include hot flashes, fatigue, decreased erectile ability, decreased sexual libido, breast tenderness, loss of bone mass, loss of muscle mass, decreased mental acuity, and risk for development of hormonally induced metabolic disorders such as diabetes or cardiovascular diseases. Some of these side effects clearly affect quality of life, although others may affect one's clinical health as well. It may be difficult to alleviate many of the side effects associated with hormonal therapy, since these occur because of the withdrawal of the male hormone testosterone that is required for so many aspects of a man's health. It would be inconceivable to replace a man's hormones that would otherwise exacerbate his advanced prostate cancer condition.

CHEMOTHERAPY

Chemotherapy for advanced prostate cancer carries potential side effects as well. Chemotherapy drugs are known to produce nausea and vomiting. Several antinausea medications are available and can help control this problem. Hair loss may also occur as a side effect of chemotherapy. It can also affect the formation of circulating blood cells and platelets. This effect may result from the toxicity of chemotherapy on bone marrow, the source of circulating blood cells. The loss of blood cells may make a person anemic, susceptible to infection, or at risk for bleeding. Transfusion of blood products may be necessary to offset these complications. Chemotherapy may also cause diarrhea because of the effect of such drugs on the lining of the intestine. It is important for you to drink enough fluids to prevent dehydration, and your physician may also prescribe medication to help slow the diarrhea. Sores in the mouth and throat can also occur because of the toxic effects of chemotherapy drugs. Ice chips, lip balm, and gargling may relieve these symptoms, but your doctor may need to treat severe sores with medicine.

SUMMARY

Side effects from treatment of prostate cancer do occur and must be balanced against the effectiveness of various treatments. Knowledge of the side effects may influence the selection of the ideal treatment for you. It is important to decide which functional side effects you are most comfortable with and which risks you would rather avoid altogether.

CHAPTER 5

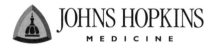

STRAIGHT TALK—
COMMUNICATION WITH
FAMILY, FRIENDS, AND
COWORKERS

Coming to terms with your prostate cancer diagnosis is certainly daunting. Your situation is likely similar to that of any person who is told that he has a significant disease state or cancer diagnosis. Often, the reaction upon hearing the prostate cancer diagnosis is complete shock and bewilderment. Emotions block out any kind of rational thinking much of the time. Further feelings of "how can this happen to me?" certainly are normal. After being shocked by the news, additional feelings of self-pity, sadness, and even hopelessness surface.

It is important to understand that these emotions are normal. At the same time, the next step is action in coping with the diagnosis, which includes not only you but all of those surrounding you including family, friends, and co-workers. In addition to your adjustment to having this diagnosis, the communication and interaction with many around you is also extremely important. Most persons will feel anxious or embarrassed by your diagnosis. Keeping those around you informed in a way that allows them to deal with it constructively and to give you positive support will be most helpful to you. Some thoughts are provided here to begin to produce a constructive environment and achieve positive communication with various persons involved in your life.

SHARING YOUR CANCER DIAGNOSIS

Understandably, emotions will be heavily charged upon learning of a cancer diagnosis for anyone. A great deal of anxiety can be expected in beginning to understand the facts of your disease and in making decisions about how you wish to proceed with medical management. Amid these practical concerns, the concern of one's own personal adjustment to the diagnosis is critical. An initial step in the process of coping clearly is to admit to yourself how you feel. Each individual needs to understand his own personality and how he reacts to challenging circumstances in life. You may have to identify appropriately positive coping mechanisms that work for you. Initial reactions may include denial and embarrassment and perhaps a sense that you do not want to discuss the matter much with anyone. However, as time moves forward, it may be useful to consider how and when you would like to talk to your spouse or significant other, other family members, and possibly particular friends about having a prostate cancer diagnosis.

Most people do need and want to talk to someone. Loved ones can certainly be your sounding board as you begin to take in the reality of your situation. These individuals should certainly be supportive of you, and by talking with them you may be able to better solve your problems and sort our issues that have mounted relating to your prostate cancer diagnosis. Close friends and family should certainly know you best—your personality and the way you handle things—to provide the very best assistance during this difficult time. You may also find that as you begin to share your diagnosis several individuals around you may come forward to acknowledge their bouts with cancer and how they were able to cope in different ways. A bond may form in a very special way with another individual or two who may also have prostate cancer and are making decisions themselves for moving forward with any form of treatment for it.

JUGGLING UNEXPECTED FEELINGS

Friends and family members surrounding you may react in different ways upon hearing your diagnosis. Some may be sobered by the news that you have cancer and may not know how to approach you. It can be expected that all loving family members and friends do wish to support you, but they may not know how. Though positive support can generally be expected, almost unexpectedly negative reactions can also occur. Family members may struggle to be supportive upon knowing that their own life circumstances may be disrupted to help you with your needs. A certain feeling of resentment may come upon an individual who knows that he/she will have to take some responsibilities for you while also dealing with his/her own personal and professional capacities. Even when family members appear quite pleasant and supportive, they may still have some sense of anger and, unfortunately, express these feelings at times toward you. It is important to keep in mind that this response is not directed specifically toward you but likely the entire situation, and thus you should not feel at fault. It is also important to recognize that many people react differently to stressful situations depending upon their own personal experiences and personalities. You should not be alarmed if family members become somewhat depressed themselves and react in different ways, such as becoming more absorbed in work or engaging in activities outside the home. Other family members may become more attentive to you but overly involved in such a way that reflects their possible depression and sense of guilt. The best reaction for all is to be honest about how they feel. Constructive action can be taken afterward for various individuals to interact most appropriately for both you and them.

DISCUSSING YOUR FEARS

Upon learning of your diagnosis, you may feel a certain amount of fear and anxiety. Others around you may also express these same feelings. Being open and honest and discussing these fears and concerns is likely to be most useful to deal with the situation. Perhaps the best strategy for dealing with fears is to become informed as much as possible about your disease state and then have loving members of your family and friends help you sort through the information you need to know. Once you are more informed, many fears are conquered. Though you may be frightened to consider the prospect of your disease state, treatments that could be offered to you, and any potential side effects or changes in your life associated with treatments, quite commonly many fears abate when answers become available for any frightening concerns you may have.

FINDING YOUR OWN VOICE

Conversations about having a prostate cancer diagnosis are never easy. You certainly may be uncomfortable presenting any concerns that you have. Your supporters may also struggle in expressing all concerns. There is no right way to handle any of this. Rather, you may decide when and how to begin any sort of conversation. At the same time, you may want individuals around you just to be sounding boards, willing to listen to your concerns without passing any sort of judgment or advice.

Understandably, not everyone immediately surrounding you has the capability to respond to you in the most constructive way or in a way that you believe will help you cope. Support groups may be very helpful in this regard. Support may come from participating in various workshops, peer groups, or religious groups. Such an organization is Us TOO, a self-help support group for prostate cancer survivors and their families. Another support group, called Man to Man, is also available for support and information. Support groups may also be extremely advantageous by offering interactions with individuals who may currently have or had previously dealt with a prostate cancer diagnosis. Any such individual may certainly know exactly what you are going through and can offer support in ways that those who have not encountered the diagnosis would be unable to do. Support may be simply a matter of having a trusted individual who can listen well and be supportive.

Beyond these support mechanisms, you may wish to communicate with select individuals using a diary or journal to avoid having to repeat yourself many times about your own progress. In this modern era of the Internet, you may explore using a Web site or "blog" that can be accessed by cancer patients and families for updating medical information regularly without having to distribute the information exhaustively to different individuals about your progress. These examples all suggest that there are various mechanisms and resources that can be applied to be communicative. You may decide to apply any one of these or perhaps multiple resources. It is all up to you.

TALKING WITH YOUNG CHILDREN ABOUT YOUR CANCER

It is one thing to communicate the many aspects of your prostate cancer diagnosis to your adult relatives, but having to communicate this life situation to young children in your life can be particularly challenging. It is understandable that you do not wish to inform them about your prostate cancer diagnosis early, if at all, to hide any sort of fears or worries associated with the diagnosis from them. At some point, however, it may be appropriate to disclose the diagnosis of your prostate cancer so they will be able to adjust most effectively. Children can be very perceptive and may appreciate that something is wrong. In addition, if they witness any changes in your life or your physical appearance, they may suspect something is wrong. It may be better to enlighten them so they can cope appropriately and not derive any sort of misconceptions.

More than likely, your ability to discuss the matter with children will occur after many of your strong emotions have passed. You may decide what information and how much information to share once you are much more familiar with your own condition. Much as you may be confused and unclear about the meaning of cancer and its impact on your life, children will undoubtedly be affected in similar ways, although they may not be able to voice their concerns to you or others as well. Explanations that are accurate but appropriate for their level of understanding will certainly help them deal with the news of your prostate cancer diagnosis. Basic concepts without too many abstract meanings are fundamentally helpful. You may be able to convey to them a positive way of handling the situation so that their fears and anxieties can be allayed.

It is important to try to maintain a "normal" routine and lifestyle for children. However, they should certainly be prepared for any changes that may happen in the family. They may become depressed by any thought of death or separation of a family member. If you have any sense that a child in your life is taking the situation extremely hard and may benefit from professional help, action should be taken to be sure he/she is supported as well. Professional help may be required, and a social worker or school psychologist may be enlisted to talk with your child. Support groups also exist for children, and it may be extremely important to find these as a resource for support outside of the family.

TELLING YOUR ADULT CHILDREN AND PARENTS

Adult family members, particularly older individuals such as parents, may also struggle upon learning of your prostate cancer diagnosis. Unlike children, they may not have fictional concerns, but they may be equally irrational about knowing how to deal with the situation. Adult children may become emotional when realizing the impact of a parent's cancer diagnosis. They may realize how important you are to them and possibly experience guilt because of any separation they have had in the past. They may feel remorseful because they are unable to spend a lot of time with you because of living far away or having employment obligations. Adult children may become even more protective and want to know everything about your management to ensure that you are receiving the very best care.

Parents may also struggle with an adult child's prostate cancer diagnosis. Parents may be older and in relatively poor health limiting their physical, mental, and perhaps emotional ability to handle your life situation. The idea that their child carries a cancer diagnosis may be particularly hard on them. Finding ways to discuss the matter with them where they can feel included and informed without creating more stress for them makes sense. Support groups and other resources may also be useful to them.

INFORMING YOUR FRIENDS

Having friends in your life has been important to support you throughout good and bad times. They have been your allies. It can be expected that they would be supportive of you through the tough time of having a prostate cancer diagnosis. The decision to discuss your diagnosis with friends remains yours alone. But sharing your problem with people you sense will be supportive should enable you to move forward with the situation.

It is important to consider how your friends may respond to you upon learning of your prostate cancer diagnosis. Before you talk to others about your illness, you may wish to think through your own feelings, your reasons for telling them, and your expectations of them. It is often the case that people do not know what to say, which makes them feel awkward and uncomfortable. They may feel that it is easier to say nothing because they fear they may say the wrong thing. Some may indeed become withdrawn or distance themselves from you. This reaction may actually extend from a fear of possibly losing you. Other close friends may become overly considerate or intrusive. They may feel it is important to show their concern by being as helpful to you as possible. Your reaction may well be to understand all the ways your friends could react and accept their emotions and responses. Your friends should be informed by you as to how you wish for them to help you. An honest line of communication for these relationships will also be the best policy. Doing so will make it easier for them to be supportive and remain included in your life.

BALANCING NEW RELATIONSHIPS

For a single man having a prostate cancer diagnosis, maintaining a life in all respects can be especially challenging. The range of emotions is heightened because this cancer diagnosis may affect sexuality and intimacy. Prostate cancer management may affect one's sexual function directly or indirectly by changing other aspects of pelvic function including urinary and ejaculatory abilities or routines. You may have already handled your prostate cancer diagnosis adequately but find that the side effects of treatment have significantly affected your quality of life. You may have already accepted these changes or have applied urological treatments to address them to remain functional. Despite this, bodily functions can change with management of prostate cancer, and those men affected will have to decide how to make adjustments and communicate their body's changes effectively with their mate. The issue may indeed be much more acute if this person is new in your life and you are considering how to date in an open and honest way. You may have to judge when is the best time to share this part of your life with this person. It may be something to discuss once it is clear that a strong bond has been made and the person may be able to understand what you have encountered. A supportive individual will accept the truth and look to continue to develop a loving relationship.

LETTING YOUR BOSS AND COWORKERS KNOW

Informing individuals in your work environment regarding a health condition can be tricky. There may be worries that not all individuals will be in any way supportive of you and perhaps some may look to take advantage of the situation for their own personal gain. There may be worries that your having a major health condition may seriously affect your ability to perform work, and your boss may give you little consideration in this regard. You may be even more worried that your boss may look to advance assignments or extend promotions to others, and possibly relieve you of responsibilities, upon hearing of your illness.

You are not actually required to tell your boss you have cancer. Any absences can be explained by the fact that you are under a doctor's care that may require some time away from work. The Americans with Disabilities Act provides you some job protection so that arrangements can be made for you to work on a schedule that meets the medical needs of your treatment. You are also not required to provide prognostic information, information about how well you will recover and when you may be able to return to work. Again, this is your personal choice. In the end, some communication with appropriate individuals in your work environment may be necessary to define your work absence and expectations about your transition back to work in a fair and appropriate manner.

SUMMING UP: SHARING YOUR THOUGHTS AND FEELINGS ABOUT CANCER

Having cancer is hard to deal with alone. The condition evokes thoughts of powerlessness and hopelessness, so much so that individuals around you would seem unlikely to offer much help. More than likely, the truth is that many supportive individuals around you exist and can help you with dealing with this tough life situation. Steps taken to communicate your diagnosis with others and to gain their support are a very important coping strategy for you. Although talking about your cancer can be hard at first, most patients find that being honest and communicative about their cancer is most advantageous.

- *Choose a good listener.*

- *Select an appropriate time to share.*

- *Recognize your own anger or frustrations.*

- *Be honest about your emotions.*

- *Use additional community resources if feeling overwhelmed.*

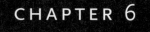

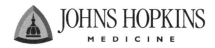
JOHNS HOPKINS
MEDICINE

Maintaining Balance—
Work and Life
During Treatment

**HELPFUL HINTS ON HOW TO PLAN CARE AND
MINIMIZE DISRUPTIONS IN YOUR LIFE**

As you prepare to undergo treatment for prostate cancer, your life will change. It is important to prepare for the requirements of your treatment and understand what life changes may be necessary, both in your personal and professional life activities. You may be accustomed to a full life with many responsibilities that will now have to be changed because of the time needed to undergo your treatment. It is important to understand and accept these changes. You may need to make adjustments in your commitments and otherwise ask people in your life, including family members and friends, to help you in different ways. All of this may seem very stressful for you and others surrounding you, but for all to understand how your life has changed is important. Look to receive their support while discussing with them frankly how they can be helpful to you.

Although your schedule may change significantly based on the need for treatment, you may wish to accept that others also have life routines to meet, particularly young children in your life. To not disrupt their activities too much, you may need to request other adult individuals in your life to step in. Again, do not be afraid to accept the help of family members, friends, and neighbors. As they aid you at this time of need, you may find a great willingness to help them in such a way some time in the future.

In preparation for treatment, you may consider various ways to plan ahead effectively. By considering how treatment for your prostate cancer may change your lifestyle at least temporarily, you may wish to plan ahead and organize how these changes will affect family members and others around you. For instance, as you plan for a surgery, you may recognize that others around you may have to help you with activities of daily living during your recuperation. Prior to your surgery date, you may wish to discuss with family members how they can help you with your recovery and what basic necessities will be needed when you return home from surgery. With proper planning, you should be able to have a comfortable surrounding in your home and accomplish simple matters such as having food in the refrigerator and clean clothes to wear. You may also wish to plan for an environment that facilitates your optimal recovery with any other comforts that suit you.

Counselors will certainly be able to advise you about what to expect with your treatment and recovery. Your physician may direct you to a patient advocate, a health center nurse, or even a social worker who may be able to help you plan ahead for your experience. Patients who have previously undergone prostate cancer treatment may be able to tell you exactly what to expect with treatment and recovery. Your treating physician should give you guidelines for your recovery in advance. You may receive some basic instructions while you may also wish to pursue further questions to be clear about considerations for recovery. You should be very familiar with even the most basic concerns of diet and activity levels postoperatively. It is important to know what your limitations should be as well as what sort of recovery exercises or routines should be pursued to enable you to recover as quickly and safely as possible.

If you are undergoing surgery, you should obtain information as necessary regarding plans for hospitalization and recovery upon returning home. You should have a good sense of when you can resume various activities including physical exercise and when you can resume full levels of work. If you are undergoing radiation, you may also be best informed regarding any plans for hospitalization or outpatient management. If radiation is to continue for several weeks, long range plans are necessary to understand how the treatment will fit in with various other life activities you may have and how these other activities may be disrupted. Radiation therapy conducted with an outpatient regimen may allow you to continue a work schedule of some sort although it may also affect your strength level and lead you to limit the number of activities you may have earlier performed. You may wish to work in some additional time on a daily basis for your personal needs and even just to rest.

CONTINUING WORK

As mentioned, for radiation treatments, many men may elect to continue with some level of work. Your schedule may have to be changed in this case. Understandably, you would want to continue to feel productive and make contributions. You may wish to continue to feel at ease in the surrounding of supportive coworkers and not spend every waking moment thinking about your cancer situation. A wise move may be to sit down with your boss and plan out a schedule that works for both of you. You may know in advance what kind of work schedule is permissible and then devise a work schedule accordingly. You may wish to schedule your radiation treatments early in the day or toward the end of the day so that you will be well enough to carry out a reasonably productive several hours of work along the way. Bosses know the importance of being flexible, and they should be supportive of you as you earnestly arrange your schedule. You are protected to some degree by the Family and Medical Leave Act as you proceed.

WHEN I MIGHT EXPECT NOT TO FEEL WELL

Side effects are well known possibilities to be associated with treatments for prostate cancer. For surgery, it would be expected that basic recovery and recuperation will occur within several weeks, or less. However, some men may struggle with regaining stamina, and they may require several additional weeks to regain enough strength for full levels of activity. In a similar way, the recovery of urinary control will be a major issue for many men. It is understandable that most men will require urinary pads or diapers during their recovery periods. Most men should expect to regain urinary continence in time. You may find that you will require pads for social decency even when resuming work. This is not unusual at all. As your body recovers and your urinary sphincter regains strength, full continence is achieved by many men within three months after their surgeries.

Similar adverse health considerations can also be expected from prostate cancer radiation therapy. It is common for men to experience a sense of fatigue while undergoing radiation, and this may become more pronounced after several weeks of such treatments. Do not be alarmed. In planning ahead, you may wish to arrange for personal time for rest. After your radiation treatments are completed, stamina will return.

INFECTION PREVENTION

As for any cancer, treatments used for prostate cancer can weaken your immune system. The treatments themselves have already weakened your body from a physical point of view. If your immune system is further compromised by your general medical conditions or the effects of treatment, you may be more susceptible to getting a cold, flu, or other form of infection.

To remain as healthy as possible, you may wish to follow some recommendations to limit any further setback with a common communicable illness. When you are particularly weakened by treatment it is wise to avoid young children who may carry infectious organisms and be sick, even when they do not act like they are. Rest as much as possible to feel well. Maintaining a balanced diet, rich in fruits and vegetables, may help to boost your immune system. For those men being treated with chemotherapy, stringent efforts should be taken to preserve the health of your immune system. In addition to basic precautions, you may elect to wear a mask in certain risky situations such as being in close quarters with sick children or traveling in closed compartments of a train or airplane. A nurse working with you during your chemotherapy treatments may further advise you regarding precautions, and inform you when you may be particularly at risk for infection. This will allow you to take the necessary safety precautions to enjoy your activites and encounters.

CHAPTER 7

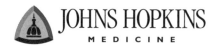

SURVIVING PROSTATE CANCER— RE-ENGAGING IN MIND–BODY HEALTH AFTER TREATMENT

SURVIVORSHIP

Surviving prostate cancer is hardly a trivial process. You may feel a sense of relief to have moved forward in a timely fashion with an effective treatment. You may have already had appropriate early clinical follow-up visits with all indicators suggesting that your disease has been eradicated. When do you consider yourself to be a survivor? The most common definition of survivorship is actually the moment you are diagnosed and have chosen to embark on a well-formulated treatment. However, the further implication is that your treatment has effectively taken care of your disease and you should have a low or virtually nonexistent likelihood of cancer recurrence. Concern about your cancer recurring and feeling anxious about this possibility is well understood. You may have given significant energies —mentally, physically, and emotionally—to fighting your disease, and lessening this fight just because your treatment has been completed may seem hard to grasp. Even after being told that your treatment was successful, you may be apprehensive about the possibility of recurrence despite acknowledging this fact on a rational level.

For many men, early diagnosis of prostate cancer means that they will be cured and stay cured with effective treatment. However, because treatment does not guarantee success and because you may be aware of men with recurrences despite the very best execution of treatment, fear and worry are usual reactions. Your doctor will certainly have advised you to continue with a surveillance program for early identification of recurrence if such a situation arises. You may understand the importance of continuing to be vigilant about this possibility and look to promote your very best health. Many men remain actively involved in their surveillance programs, which is a tribute to them. Continuing to be informed about their own health status and to keep up with the latest research developments and therapies for the field can be empowering. As you regain your physical strength, all approaches that also enable you to get back on track mentally and emotionally are most appropriate. Understand that the recovery process is not as instantaneous as completing the treatment program, and adapting at all levels of mind–body health is a natural part of the recovery process.

COUNSELING

For some patients, finding your own way to recovery is not easy, even after successful treatment. Others may experience continued distress if there is any sense that the treatment was not completely effective and that more intervention may indeed be necessary. Professional support to help you with your emotional state sometimes can be very helpful. Your surgeon or radiation therapist may be able to guide you, but their expertise is chiefly in executing treatment. A medical oncologist may offer a certain level of support, but his/her abilities as a psychological counselor may be limited. Do not be surprised if your doctor or nurse recommends that you consider seeing a trained professional counselor whose expertise and experience may be beneficial to you. A therapist of this sort may easily complement the care your other physicians provide. Such a person can be a sounding board for you to air your thoughts, and to help you gain perspective on how to deal with your situation so that you can move forward in life.

Counseling may also include hearing about the experiences of others who have been diagnosed and treated for prostate cancer. Indeed, these individuals may be advocates, survivors themselves, who support those who have followed them in their battle with cancer. They may fully understand the challenges and concerns of being a prostate cancer survivor and be able to relate their best strategies for dealing with any adversity and gaining control of one's life. You may learn from them, at a minimum, that what you are experiencing is not unique to you and rather may be a common experience of many prostate cancer survivors.

MANAGING LONG TERM SIDE EFFECTS
OF TREATMENT

One of the costs of treatment includes the possibility of physical side effects that may linger for some time. Some side effects are directly associated with the course of a treatment, and many of these should resolve once the treatment is completed. This is not always the case for cancer treatments. For prostate cancer, treatment may indeed have altered your bodily structure resulting in physical changes that may take some time to recover and possibly may never do so completely.

Some physical changes may indeed be permanent as a consequence of receiving effective treatment. Understandable early physical side effects include fatigue, weakness, trouble concentrating, and possibly even generalized aches and pains. No doubt surgery for prostate removal exerts a major impact on the body, thus requiring time for physical recuperation. Radiation therapy also causes physical effects including malaise and fatigue that may carry on through the course of treatment and persist for some time after treatment has ceased. Both localized treatments, surgery and radiation, are associated with impairments in urinary control, defecation, and sexual ability that may persist as long-term complications. Hormonal therapy or other therapies for advanced disease are well associated with side effects for the long term. In these cases, ongoing symptoms of weight gain, hot flashes, night sweats, decreased physical strength, breast tenderness, decreased sexual libido, and even changes in mental acuity are common. To proceed ahead realistically, you should have some sense of awareness of side effects that may persist after treatment and require you to adjust accordingly (see Chapter 4 for management of side effects).

LIVING A HEALTHIER LIFESTYLE

Taking charge of your health and psychological well-being should be a priority for you now. Sensible good-health recommendations are to eat healthier, maintain physical fitness, avoid physical and emotional stress, and limit exposure to unhealthful habits. The discussion below provides some helpful ways to accomplish these endeavors and feel good doing it.

> *Nutrition:* It stands to reason that if you eat
> healthier and watch your weight, you may better
> reduce your risk of prostate cancer recurrence.
> In support of this conventional wisdom, there
> is evidence that individuals who are overweight
> or obese carry more threatening risks of the
> biological progression and incurability of prostate
> cancer. To reduce the risk of prostate cancer
> recurring, many experts advocate a healthy
> diet equivalent to the diet recommended to
> keep your heart healthy. This is a diet rich in
> fruits and vegetables and limited in high fats.
> These recommendations do not preclude an
> occasional splurge to eat your favorite food or a
> treat that may have lesser dietary value. Rather,
> the recommendation is to recognize how eating
> healthier in general may give you the best long-
> term benefits. Dietary changes may indeed
> represent a lifestyle adjustment that increases

your overall fitness by way of steady and controlled weight loss. You may find that such adjustment is hard to do, but do not give up. All efforts can be expected to keep you healthy for a long time.

Exercise: Another recommendation that may help reduce the risk of prostate cancer recurrence is to establish a physical exercise regimen in your life. Finding an exercise program that works for you, and that you can commit to, should enable you to feel good about your physical well-being. Simply enough, you may just feel better to be physically in shape.

There are many different ways to be fit, and you may pursue any number of physical fitness programs that suit you. Some individuals may design and implement a training program at a local fitness center or with physical training equipment in their own homes. Others may engage in specialized activities from power walking to line dancing. The key is to identify a program that works for you by way of how your body handles the physical activity and maintains your interest. The idea is that this physical exercise program will be yours to follow for a long time and become another life adjustment. You may have to consider how to make time in your busy schedule for regular physical exercise so that it can be sustained.

Stress: Life can be stressful. Demands from work, family responsibilities, and pursuing your own personal goals may all lead to physical and emotional turmoil. Although a "don't worry, be happy" guide sounds nice, this existence may be more a fantasy than a reality for most of us. As you have undergone treatment for prostate cancer, stress was naturally associated with this process. Now that treatment is over, the new phase of your life may include resumption of chaotic life stressors. One approach to dealing with stress is to identify factors associated with it and take constructive steps to eliminate or reduce these. This adjustment may mean making some serious life adjustments. The extent of your work such as changing from a full-time to a part-time status may also be considered. Changes in your home environment may also be necessary if this will help you regain control and reduce stress in your life. Other actions may simply be to take a whole new perspective regarding what constitutes stress in your life. Having had prostate cancer, you may discover what is important and what is so unimportant that you should not have any sort of stress about it. You may quickly decide that such minor things as inconvenient appointments, delayed reports to you, and even unpleasantness of people you encounter daily should not lead you to become physically or emotionally upset. You may identify and focus on any number of joys in your life that keep you happy and maintain your emotional balance. Additional stress-relieving activities such as yoga classes or performing other forms of relaxation therapy can be useful.

Avoid smoke and alcohol: Your overall wellness program may benefit from reducing or eliminating all behaviors that compromise your best health status. Some behaviors are well known to be counterproductive to maintaining good health. Such behaviors include cigarette smoking and excessive alcohol use. Cigarette smoking is a well-known adverse health habit. The effects of cigarette smoking on inducing or promoting cancer of various forms are documented in the medical literature. Exposure to cigarette smoke may come not just by first-hand use but also secondarily by being in the environment of others who are smokers. Discontinuing cigarette smoking exposure is wise advice. Excessive alcohol use adversely affects the metabolism of the body and contributes to decreased immune health. Avoiding this risk is an action well worth taking.

SETTING NEW GOALS

Being a survivor after prostate cancer treatment means that you will continue on with life and have a future ahead of you. Your ordeal may have left you with some life adjustments to make, but you nonetheless may be prepared to move forward at this time to begin life anew. Having prostate cancer may have given you a new perspective. You may see and do things in different ways than you did previous to your prostate cancer diagnosis and treatment. This is not uncommon. Many men have reassessed their lives in the face of prostate cancer and acknowledge that life is not to be lived forever. They may have accepted their own mortality but want to move forward redefining how they want to live in the most meaningful way possible. This reassessment may give new meaning to a number of life activities that before were not so highly valued. Particular meaning may be given to rebuilding relationships and spending more time with family. Further direction may well be to set new goals in life. These goals may range from taking on that hobby that has seemed to be eternally on hold to finishing the educational degree that you had always hoped to achieve. You may find new ways to give you a sense of achievement and fulfillment. Volunteering your knowledge and experience, in settings ranging from youth programs to community service activities to participation in patient advocacy groups, may bring you enormous self-fulfillment. You may believe that such volunteer activities would allow you to leave your mark on this world or simply give you pleasure and gratification.

SEEING THE WORLD THROUGH DIFFERENT EYES

Overcoming cancer is a wondrous thing. Beating the odds and living is an almost indescribable experience. The world may appear quite different to those who have faced and grappled with cancer, and now, having overcome their diagnosis, prepare to move on in life. Prostate cancer is a life-altering condition. Once becoming a prostate cancer survivor, you may have a whole new perspective about what is important in life and what should be cherished. No doubt you are not the same person as you were before your diagnosis. Having had this diagnosis, you may find that the most remarkable and rewarding activity is to give back in some way so that other men can benefit from your experience. When you participate in prostate cancer organizations you can help men take steps to undergo screening for prostate cancer, and, if they are diagnosed, to receive proper treatment early and effectively. Any role in this process you provide is a major contribution in the fight against prostate cancer.

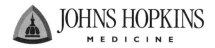

CHAPTER 8

MANAGING RISK— WHAT IF MY CANCER COMES BACK?

As for all cancers, the recurrence of prostate cancer even with the most effective curative intervention is always feared. This worry is hardly surprising. It cannot always be eliminated, but various steps should be taken to monitor yourself so that you can consider early action if the possibility of recurrence arises.

PREVENTION AND MONITORING FOR RECURRENCE

The management of prostate cancer can take various forms. Though effective treatment can be pursued once the cancer diagnosis is made, additional strategies to deal with prostate cancer should always be considered. Prevention is always the ultimate intervention; there is no better way to reduce the effects of cancer than to keep it from occurring in the first place. Prevention is the basis for the efforts of many scientists and specialists in this field. Their work will continue. Along the way, recommendations can be given to reduce the recurrence of prostate cancer after initial treatment by means of secondary prevention. You may be inclined to consider what steps to take to reduce prostate cancer recurrence. Current thought in this field suggests that secondary prevention is an appropriate action, despite the fact that the success of such action remains to be shown definitively.

Prostate cancer incidence has been associated with environmental factors such as certain environmental exposures and the diet we eat. It would then seem reasonable to strongly suggest that patients who have been diagnosed with and treated for prostate cancer adopt lifestyle changes to reduce any possible recurrence of the disease. For instance, the high fat, low vegetable and fruit diet of the Western world is believed to be a definite culprit for the development of prostate cancer. Recommended dietary changes include the intake of more fruits and vegetables and less red meat. Increased exercise to burn off calories is also recommended. These steps can reduce the fuel for any possible lingering prostate cancer cells to flourish within the body.

Excessive vitamin use, however, may be disadvantageous. The idea of using vitamins to remain healthy seems logical. Though it seems that using vitamins should improve your defenses against recurrences of prostate cancer, recent studies have offered some evidence that excessive vitamin use may actually promote cancer progression. The take-home message would be to use vitamins at recommended dosages, eat a healthy diet, and maintain a physical activity regimen as your primary prevention activities. These recommendations may sound familiar if you have heard recommendations to maintain cardiovascular health. Simply said, a good diet and exercise plan may preserve good health not just for your heart and circulatory system but also for your prostate.

The recurrence of prostate cancer may become a reality for some men despite receiving effective treatment. The risk for recurrence depends upon a number of factors. These include issues relating to the characteristics of the initial prostate cancer diagnosis and the effectiveness of treatment. These features include the aggressiveness level of the cancer (also known as grade) and the extent of progression (also known as stage) at the time of treatment. We know that men with favorable prostate cancer presentations of low grade and early stage do well, and are unlikely to have a recurrence. In contrast, men who have very aggressive prostate cancer are at greater risk for recurrence. For this group, there is a risk of cancer progression in the vicinity of the prostate, even when effective surgery or radiation has been given. In men who have undergone surgery, pathologic processing of the removed prostate and seminal vesicles along with lymph nodes can aid in gauging the success of the surgery and for predicting risk of recurrence. Pathological features from the surgical specimens can be prognostic. In addition to a final determination of the cancer's grade to be at the high range of Gleason scores (8-10), finding cancer at the surgical margins, invading the seminal vesicles, or spread to lymph nodes, informs the surgeon of an adverse situation. This information can then be shared with patients so that they can decide upon the need for further action. Sometimes immediate further therapies such as radiation to follow surgery can be implemented for high-risk situations. Standard observation may also be appropriate in situations where a low risk likelihood of recurrence exists. Your surgeon should thoroughly discuss with you what sort of risk profile can be estimated and how further management should proceed following a radical prostatectomy. Similarly, for men undergoing primary radiation therapy, the radiation oncologist should counsel you further regarding your risk profile.

Standard monitoring should be performed after effective localized treatment in everybody, including men thought to be at low risk for prostate cancer recurrence. Since prostate cancer can recur in even the most favorable circumstances, there are no exceptions to this recommendation. There is no reason that any man should not be closely monitored after receiving initial treatment. An additional consideration is that the early identification of any sort of recurrence allows the initiation of further therapy when it is likely to be most useful and effective. This monitoring is generally quite easily done by using the PSA test. This approach involves blood testing for this chemical marker at scheduled time points after initial treatment. Depending upon whether surgery or radiation was carried out, the PSA level will be absent or hardly measurable—with radiation the prostate is not removed from the body, and a low level measurement that does not rise still means that the cancer is under control. After surgery or radiation therapy, PSA monitoring is extremely sensitive and specific, and it is usually the best way to know whether the cancer remains sufficiently controlled. It is certainly better than tracking any sort of symptoms of prostate cancer recurrence or performing physical examinations or radiographic imaging in hopes of picking up recurrences early. Simply stated, with serial monitoring the PSA will rise (or change to become measurable) well in advance of other techniques that could be used to detect recurrences. This does not mean that other monitoring techniques cannot be applied along the way. These can be performed, although PSA testing is the major basis for monitoring disease recurrence.

If a PSA change occurs following treatment, this may be the first sign of prostate cancer recurrence. Sometimes a repeat test to be sure that the change has occurred is performed. This is recommended because sometimes an error in measurement is made in the laboratory. Once the PSA change is verified, an assessment of your options for further management should be done with your doctor. This assessment encompasses a review of your original prostate cancer diagnosis and management, the time frame by which your PSA measurement has now become measurable or changed, and goals for further management in the context of your overall current health condition. PSA changes within the first two years of initial treatment are more indicative of a high-risk prostate cancer recurrence than a change that occurs many years following treatment. Your doctor may understand your threat of prostate cancer recurrence better by checking it a few additional times (over months) after the initial change. If the PSA increases are observed to be minimal, prostate cancer recurrence is likely to be a low threat. On the other hand, if the PSA increases on repeated checks are rapidly elevating, a more threatening prostate cancer recurrence is generally suspected. To help with defining the recurrence, radiographic imaging studies may be ordered at this time. These may include bone scans, CAT scans, prostascint, or other scans. Your doctor will decide which scans are most appropriate for this purpose.

A radiographic finding indicating prostate cancer spread will focus disease management decision making on advanced prostate cancer. Because prostate cancer often recurs after other health problems have developed, it is important to consider whether the patient's overall health condition could influence the risks or benefits of further prostate cancer treatment. The complete picture may suggest that the threat of the prostate cancer is a low priority with respect to the patient's other health conditions. Because prostate cancer progresses slowly in many instances, appropriate treatment should be given only if the threat of the prostate cancer progressing and limiting survival is high. Conservative management with clinical monitoring may be appropriate for many men. All of these issues warrant thorough discussion This discussion may include not just your treating urologist or radiation oncologist, but a medical oncologist or other advanced prostate cancer specialists (see Chapter 10).

TREATMENT OPTIONS
(LOCAL VS. DISTANT RECURRENCE)

Based on the confirmation of a prostate cancer recurrence and the life-threatening risk, this management ranging from conservative monitoring to active additional therapy can be considered. Active treatment is appropriate for the man at risk for rapid prostate cancer progression and death from his disease. For a man who was managed initially with radical prostatectomy, a local recurrence (cancer progression in the vicinity of the prostate) may prompt consideration for salvage radiation therapy to the pelvic region. A distant recurrence (cancer progression beyond the pelvic region) in the man initially treated by radical prostatectomy would not likely be suitable for radiation therapy. Advanced prostate cancer is best treated by hormonal therapy or other treatments for advanced prostate cancer. A local recurrence in the man initially treated by radiation therapy usually can not be treated with further radiation because of the risk of radiation-induced complications. Hormonal therapy is commonly administered in the instance of radiation failure. Alternative options for suspected local recurrence after radiation failure include salvage radical prostatectomy and cryosurgery. These alternatives should be carefully considered in light of their investigational nature and the fact that they are associated with high complication risks. If the radiation failure is believed to be associated with the distant spread of disease, standard hormonal therapy is the option of choice. Chemotherapeutic options may also be applied in settings of distant recurrences following either surgery or radiation, and these options can be discussed further with an advanced prostate cancer specialist or medical oncologist.

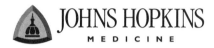

CHAPTER 9

JOHNS HOPKINS

M E D I C I N E

My Cancer Isn't Curable— What Now?

UNDERSTANDING TREATMENT GOALS FOR METASTATIC DISEASE

Situations arise in which cure for prostate cancer is not possible. A man may have been diagnosed relatively late in the course of the disease process beyond which any standard localized treatment such as surgery or radiation will be effective. Another may have been diagnosed when treatment was thought to be potentially effective, but in time the cancer persists or recurs. In such instances, the prostate cancer may have spread to locations beyond the prostate indicating that the cancer has become metastatic. No doubt this is devastating news. To hear that your disease has spread beyond its site of origin and is coursing throughout the body conjures up the notion that the cancer will soon take over the body and possibly cause death.

The long-term management program will typically involve the medical oncologist. In general, advanced or metastatic prostate cancer is treated by hormonal suppression; that is, to withdraw from the body the male androgen hormone that prostate cancer cells use as a fuel to feed their growth. Hormonal therapy is not considered an approach for cure but a means of disease control. Chemotherapeutic options remain fairly minimal, and their application to prostate cancer management may come about through patient involvement in clinical trials.

Within this scope of management, men who have advanced prostate cancer must view their disease state in a different way than a man who has been successfully cured of his disease. While you and your doctor may work together to control your advanced prostate cancer, you may also want to think about your overall approach to life and what gives you the most fulfillment and quality of life.

SETTING SHORT-TERM GOALS

The setting of short-term goals is not meant to be fatalistic. It does not mean that you are giving up any sort of hope to have your disease conquered, and it should not direct you to give up on life or fail to enjoy every precious day that you have before you. The suggestion is merely to help bring focus to what is important for you to achieve your goals in a realistic manner, given the circumstances of your disease. This action coincides with organizing your personal matters such as finances, estate planning, and the like. You may have to realistically plan ahead for what you can truly accomplish and cannot accomplish with a good handle on your expected longevity. It is important to speak to your doctor frankly about what to expect from your treatment. You need to understand what your physical capacity will be during the course of these treatments, and what you should anticipate with regard to your response to them. Ask your doctor what your odds are for beating the disease and what life span you may have ahead of you. Although these discussions are hard and frightening, they are necessary for your proper life planning.

QUALITY OF LIFE VS. QUANTITY OF LIFE

Living a long life is important, but there should also be importance in the quality of one's life. When prostate cancer has metastasized, an obvious goal would be to pursue aggressive treatments that would give any man under this circumstance the most days to live. This aim is very reasonable. At the same time, it is important to consider whether advanced treatments take away from one's quality of life. Side effects are associated with hormonal therapies and chemotherapies. These therapies can cause toxic effects that may lead to a diminished quality of life; sometimes they even shorten it. You should discuss the advantages and disadvantages of all of the possible treatments with your doctor. Metastatic prostate cancer can also cause pain, especially if it has spread to bone. Living in pain clearly detracts from life's pleasures. Pain symptoms are usually associated with bone metastases, and they should always be brought to the attention of your treating doctors. Management may range from standard pain medication to specialized treatments.

For example, a painful area of metastatic prostate cancer in the back can usually be relieved by radiation therapy to the spine.

WHEN SHOULD I STOP TREATMENT?

This is not an easy question to ask of your doctor and one that is not easy for him/her to answer either. If the treatment you are receiving is proven to be ineffective and also if treatment is causing side effects without benefit, this question may arise. A frank conversation with your doctor may be necessary to gain proper perspective. The answer may be difficult to handle, just because the thought of abandoning treatment sounds like one is giving up. The matter may be tough not only on the patient but also on the physician. Physicians compassionately dispense care and take on a mission to save lives, but they may also identify when a treatment is not effective and understand when alleviating suffering must naturally occur. The time when aggressive treatments may be discontinued may indicate your need to move urgently in organizing your personal affairs and having your wishes, such as advanced directives, known prior to death.

HOSPICE/PALLIATIVE CARE

Unless life is ended abruptly by some serious event or accident, the end of life signaled by an advancing chronic disease should be handled by specialized medical services known as hospice care. Such services help in preparing for one's leaving this world, dying with dignity as well as with pain under control, and having emotional needs of the loved one's family met. Plans to seek hospice care may commonly be arranged around the time that a decision is made that treatment is no longer benefiting you. A referral from your doctor should facilitate the process. Hospice care can be arranged at a hospice facility or in your home or that of a relative. How you would like to receive this care is your choice. Your wishes should be honored as to how you desire to live toward the end of your life and to die peacefully. Additional services in the way of counseling for family members can be quite helpful. Spiritual advisors may also provide an essential role at this time.

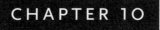

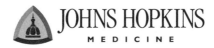

CHAPTER 10

PROSTATE CANCER IN OLDER ADULTS

by Gary R. Shapiro, MD

Prostate cancer is the leading cancer diagnosis and the second leading cause of cancer deaths among men in the United States. It is a disease of aging. As we live longer, the number of men with prostate cancer will increase dramatically. In the next 25 years, the number of people 65 years of age and older will double, and the largest increases in cancer incidence will occur in those older than 80 years of age.

If one looks for it, the vast majority of older men (over 75 years of age) have cancer cells in their prostate. The other fact is that these cells will never bother most of these men. Unlike those with other types of cancer, many men with a diagnosis of prostate cancer will never experience complications or early death from prostate cancer. Older men commonly face the dilemma of whether or not to have their prostate cancer treated. Overtreatment is common, and it is critically important that you get advice about all of your options, especially expectant management ("watchful waiting"), from a knowledgeable prostate cancer specialist. Importantly, "watchful waiting" as a form of expectant management differs from "active surveillance" as another form of expectant management. "Watchful waiting" implies a less rigorous approach to monitoring for possible disease progression and generally invokes palliative (symptom relieving) interventions when needed.

Though low-risk disease is common, a significant number of older men will have high-risk prostate cancer that should be treated aggressively. It is not always easy to know if someone's prostate cancer is high- or low-risk, but your doctor should be able to help you. Once you understand how risky your prostate cancer is, you will then need to carefully assess whether treatment will help or hurt you. Older adults with cancer often have other chronic health problems and may be taking multiple medications that can affect their cancer treatment plan. Prejudice, misunderstanding, and limited access to clinical trials often prevent older patients from getting the cancer treatment they need.

WHY IS THERE MORE CANCER IN OLDER PEOPLE?

The organs in our bodies are made up of cells. Cells divide and multiply as the body needs them. Cancer develops when cells in a part of the body grow out of control. The body has a number of ways of repairing damaged control mechanisms, but as we get older, these do not work as well. Although our healthier lifestyles have allowed us to avoid death from infection, heart attack, and stroke, we may now live long enough for a cancer to develop. People who live longer have increased exposure to cancer-causing agents (carcinogens) in the environment. Aging decreases the body's ability to protect us from these carcinogens and to repair cells that are damaged by these and other processes.

DECISION MAKING: 7 PRACTICAL STEPS

1. GET A DIAGNOSIS

No matter how "typical" the signs and symptoms, first impressions are sometimes wrong. Older men with urinary problems are more likely to have an enlarged prostate (BPH, benign prostatic hyperplasia) than high-risk prostate cancer, and a slightly elevated PSA may not be a sign of aggressive prostate cancer, either.

Though an older man with a high PSA and bone metastases is likely to have prostate cancer, he may have some other cancer in his bones and a coincidental low-risk prostate cancer. In such a case, treatment should be directed at the metastatic cancer and not the unimportant prostate cancer. A diagnosis helps you and your family understand what to expect and how to prepare for the future, even if you cannot get curative treatment. Knowing the diagnosis also helps your doctor treat your symptoms better. Many people find "not knowing" very hard and are relieved when they finally have an explanation for their symptoms. Sometimes a frail patient is obviously dying, and diagnostic studies can be an additional burden. In such cases, it may be quite reasonable to focus on symptom relief (palliation) without knowing the details of the diagnosis.

2. KNOW THE CANCER'S STAGE

The cancer's stage defines your prognosis and treatment options. No one can make informed decisions without it. Just as there may be times when the burdens of diagnostic studies may be too great, it may also be appropriate to do without full staging in a very frail, dying patient.

As in younger patients, the stage is determined by the size and extent of the tumor, the presence or absence of cancer in lymph nodes, or its spread (metastasis) to other organs. When doctors combine this information with information regarding your PSA level, cancer type, and Gleason score (see Chapter 1), they can predict what impact, if any, your prostate cancer is likely to have on your life expectancy and quality of life.

3. KNOW YOUR LIFE EXPECTANCY

Anticancer treatment should be considered if you are likely to live long enough to experience symptoms or premature death from prostate cancer. If your life expectancy is so short that the cancer will not significantly affect it, there may be no reason to treat your cancer.

However, chronological age (how old you are) should not be the only thing that decides how your cancer should, or should not, be treated. Despite advanced age, men who are relatively well often have a life expectancy that is longer than their life expectancy with prostate cancer. The average 70-year-old man is likely to live another 12 years. A similar 85-year-old can expect to live an additional five years and remain independent for most of that time. Even an unhealthy 75-year-old man probably will live five more years,

long enough to suffer symptoms and early death from metastatic prostate cancer.

4. UNDERSTAND THE GOALS

The Goals of Treatment

It is important to be clear whether the goal of treatment
is cure (surgery or radiation therapy for early stage prostate cancer) or palliation (treatment for metastatic prostate
cancer). If the goal is palliation, you need to understand if
the treatment plan will extend your life, control your symptoms, or both? How likely is it to achieve these goals, and
how long will you enjoy its benefits? Many men choose
watchful waiting (routine health monitoring) as the best
strategy for them.

When the goal of treatment is palliation, hormonal suppression or chemotherapy should never be administered
without defined endpoints and timelines. It should be clear
to everyone what "counts" as success, how it will be determined (for example, a symptom controlled or a smaller
mass on CT scan), and when. You and your family should
understand what your options are at each step and how
likely each is to meet your goals. If this is not clear, ask your
doctor to explain it in words that you understand.

The Goals of the Patient

In addition to the traditional goals of tumor response, increased survival, and symptom control, older cancer patients often have goals related to quality of life. These may
include physical and intellectual independence, spending
quality time with your family, taking trips, staying out of

89

the hospital, or even economic stability. At times, palliative care or hospice may meet these goals better than active anticancer treatment. In addition to the medical team, older patients often turn to family, friends, and clergy for guidance.

5. DETERMINE IF YOU ARE FIT OR FRAIL

Deciding how to treat cancer in someone who is older requires a thorough understanding of his general health and social situation. Decisions about cancer treatment should never focus on age alone.

Age Is Not a Number

Your actual age (chronological age) has limited influence on how cancer will respond to therapy or its prognosis. Biological and other changes associated with aging are more reliable in estimating an individual's vigor, life expectancy, or the risk of treatment complications. These changes include malnutrition, loss of muscle mass and strength, depression, dementia, falls, social isolation, and the ability to accomplish daily activities such as dressing, bathing, eating, shopping, housekeeping, and managing one's finances or medication.

Chronic Illnesses

Older cancer patients are likely to have chronic illnesses (comorbidity) that affect their life expectancy; the more that you have, the greater the effect. This effect has very little impact on the behavior of the cancer itself, but studies do show that comorbidity has a major effect on treatment outcome and its side effects.

6. BALANCE BENEFITS AND HARMS

Fit older prostate cancer patients respond to treatment similarly to their younger counterparts. However, a word of caution is in order. Until recently, few studies included very old individuals, and it may not be appropriate to apply these findings to the diverse group of older cancer patients.

The side effects of cancer treatment are never less in the elderly. In addition to the standard side effects, significant age-related toxicities must be considered. Though most of these are more a function of frailty than chronological age, even the fittest senior cannot avoid the physical effects of aging. In addition to the changes in fat and muscle that you see in the mirror, there are age-related changes in your kidney, liver, and digestive (gastrointestinal) function. These changes affect how your body absorbs and metabolizes anticancer drugs and other medicines. The average older man takes many different medicines (to control medical conditions like high blood pressure, high cholesterol, osteoporosis, diabetes, arthritis, etc.). This "polypharmacy" can cause undesirable side effects as the many drugs interact with each other and the anticancer medications.

7. GET INVOLVED

Health care providers and family members often underestimate the physical and mental abilities of older people and their willingness to face chronic and life-threatening conditions. Studies clearly show that older patients want detailed and easily understood information about potential treatments and alternatives. Patients and families may consider cancer untreatable in the aged and not understand the possibilities treatment offers.

Though patients with dementia pose a unique challenge, they are frequently capable of participating in goal setting and simple discussions about treatment side effects and logistics. Caring family members and friends are often able to share the patient's life story so that health care workers can work with them to make decisions consistent with the patient's values and desires. This of course is no substitute for a well thought out and properly executed Living Will or healthcare proxy.

Though facing the possibility of life-threatening events at any age is hard, it is always better to be prepared and to "put your affairs in order." In addition to estate planning and wills, it is critical that you outline your wishes regarding medical care at the end of life and make legal provisions for someone to make those decisions if you are unable to make them for yourself.

TREATING PROSTATE CANCER

YOU NEED A TEAM

Cancer care changes rapidly, and it is hard for the generalist to keep up to date, so referral to a specialist is essential. The needs of an older cancer patient often extend beyond the doctor's office and the traditional services visiting nurses provide. These needs may include transportation and nutritional, emotional, financial, physical, or spiritual support. When an older man with prostate cancer is the primary care giver for a frail or ill spouse, grandchildren, or other family members, special attention is necessary to provide for their needs as well. Older cancer patients cared for in geriatric oncology programs benefit from multidisciplinary teams of oncologists, geriatricians, psychiatrists, pharmacists, physiatrists, social workers, nurses, clergy, and dieticians, all working together as a team to identify and manage the stressors that can limit effective cancer treatment.

WATCHFUL WAITING

As discussed above, and in Chapter 3, many men will carry a diagnosis of prostate cancer that may not necessarily threaten their life spans. This is often the situation for older men who have a life expectancy of less than 10 years. A diagnostic work-up done when indicated in an older man may yield a prostate cancer diagnosis that will unlikely cause death with respect to the expected longevity of the patient.

Importantly, watchful waiting differs somewhat from expectant management in concept. Watchful waiting implies routine basic health monitoring either for any constitutional signs of health changes from having cancer, such as general malaise, sense of tiredness or weight loss changes, or for new urinary symptoms that may be related to locally advancing prostate cancer. Reactive interventions to maintain wellness despite the presence of cancer are generally then offered. In contrast, expectant management refers to an active surveillance program that includes regularly performed prostate examinations, PSA testing, and prostate biopsies to be able to recognize the early progression of a known low risk prostate cancer diagnosis. This rigor offers the opportunity to manage the disease in a timely way with curative intent when needed.

SURGERY

Surgery is as effective for disease eradication in elderly patients as in younger patients (see Chapter 3), but it does present a somewhat higher risk of complications in older individuals who have other medical problems (comorbidities). Radical prostatectomy in the very old is often a high-risk procedure with complications, and it is generally not advised for this group.

RADIATION THERAPY

When "watchful waiting" is not advisable, radiation therapy is an excellent option for older men with localized prostate cancer (see Chapter 3). Though studies in older men have found no significant increase in the side effects from radiation therapy, the fatigue that often accompanies radiation therapy can be quite profound in the elderly, even in those who are fit. Often the logistical details (like daily travel to the hospital for a six-week course of treatment) are the hardest for older people. It is important that you discuss these potential problems with your family and social worker before starting radiation therapy. Some older men find interstitial seed (brachytherapy) radiotherapy "easier" than external beam radiotherapy.

Radiation therapy (external beam) is particularly effective in treating bone pain caused by prostate cancer metastases to the bone. A short course of radiation therapy often allows patients with advanced cancer to lower (or even eliminate) their dose of narcotic pain relievers. Although these medicines do an excellent job of controlling pain, they often cause confusion, falls, and constipation in older patients. Thus, even hospice patients suffering from localized meta-static bone pain should consider the option of palliative radiation therapy.

HORMONAL THERAPY

Hormonal therapy (androgen deprivation therapy) is the most widely used type of treatment in prostate cancer. Usually used alone, it may be combined with radiation for localized disease. It is the cornerstone of treatment for metastatic prostate cancer. It is not unusual for men to take some form of hormonal therapy, and to live with the side effects, for the rest of their life. Older men experience these side effects (hot flashes, decreased libido, and erectile dysfunction) no less than younger men do. Additional age-related problems do, however, concern them.

Although most older men tolerate androgen deprivation therapy quite well, it can cause diabetes and cardiovascular disease, especially in those who had these problems before they started therapy. Cognitive impairment (dementia), loss of muscle mass, and osteoporosis (bone density) are particularly debilitating side effects in older men. They can cause falls and bone fractures and take away one's independence.

CHEMOTHERAPY

Nonfrail older cancer patients respond to chemotherapy similarly to their younger counterparts. Reducing the dose of chemotherapy based purely on chronological age may seriously affect the effectiveness of treatment. Managing chemotherapy-associated toxicity with appropriate supportive care is crucial in the elderly population to give them the best palliation and chance of prolonged survival.

Older men whose prostate cancers have progressed despite first-line hormonal therapy have the same benefits from docetaxel (Taxotere)-based chemotherapy as their younger counterparts. Age alone should not exclude them from receiving these or other chemotherapy regimens.

Though the side effects of cancer treatment are never less burdensome in the elderly, they can be managed by oncologists, especially geriatric oncologists, who work in teams with others who specialize in the care of the elderly. With appropriate care, healthy older patients do just as well with chemotherapy as younger patients. Advances in supportive care (antinausea medicines and blood cell growth factors) have significantly decreased the side effects of chemotherapy and have safely improved the quality of life of individuals with prostate cancer. Nonetheless, there is risk, especially if the patient is frail. The presence of severe comorbidities, age-related frailty, or underlying severe psychosocial problems may be obstacles for highly intensive treatment plans. Such patients may benefit from less complicated or potentially less toxic treatment plans.

COMMON TREATMENT COMPLICATIONS IN THE ELDERLY

Anemia (low red blood cell count) is common in the elderly, especially the frail elderly. It decreases the effectiveness of chemotherapy and often causes fatigue, falls, cognitive decline (e.g., dementia, disorientation or confusion), and heart problems. Therefore, anemia must be recognized and corrected with red blood cell transfusions or the appropriate use of erythropoiesis-stimulating agents such as epoetin (Procrit, Epogen) or darbepoetin (Aranesp).

Myelosuppression (low white blood cell count) is also common in older patients getting chemotherapy or radiation therapy. Older patients with myelosuppression develop life-threatening infections more often than younger patients, and they may need to be treated in the hospital for many days. The liberal use of granulopoietic growth factors (G-CSF, Neupogen, Neulasta) decreases the risk of infection and makes it possible for older men to receive full doses of chemotherapy.

Mucositis (mouth sores) and diarrhea can cause severe dehydration in older patients who often are already dehydrated due to inadequate fluid intake and diuretics ("water pills" for high blood pressure or heart failure). Careful monitoring and the liberal use of antidiarrheal agents (Imodium) and oral and intravenous fluids are essential components of the management of older cancer patients. Chemotherapy-induced nausea and vomiting can contribute to dehydration, and it is essential that elderly patients receive enough medicine (antiemetics) to control this.

Surgery, radiation therapy, and chemotherapy can cause other gastrointestinal side effects, including pain and obstruction. The resulting constipation can be particularly difficult to manage in elderly patients who are prone to this problem. The dehydration and poor appetite that often accompanies chemotherapy can also make constipation

97

worse. Maintaining adequate nutrition and fluid intake and careful use of stool softeners and laxatives are essential.

Kidney function declines as we age. Some of the medicines that older patients take to treat both their cancer (e.g., zoledronic acid, NSAIDs) and noncancer-related problems might make this worse. The dehydration that often accompanies cancer and its treatment can put additional stress on the kidneys. Fortunately, it is often possible to minimize these effects by carefully selecting and dosing appropriate drugs, managing "polypharmacy," and preventing dehydration.

Neurotoxicity and Cognitive Effects ("Chemo-brain") can be profoundly debilitating in patients who are already cognitively impaired (demented, disoriented, confused, etc.). Elderly patients with a history of falling, hearing loss, or peripheral neuropathy (nerve damage from, e.g., diabetes) have decreased energy and are highly vulnerable to neurotoxic chemotherapy such as the taxane compounds. Many medicines used to control nausea (antiemetics) or decrease the side effects of certain chemotherapeutic agents are also potential neurotoxins. These include ranitidine (agitation), diphenhydramine, some of the antiemetics (sedation), and dexamethasone (psychosis and agitation). The corticosteroids (prednisone, dexamethasone) are also used to treat metastatic prostate cancer.

Fatigue is a near universal complaint of older cancer patients. It is particularly a problem for those who are socially isolated or who depend upon others to help them with activities of daily living. It is not necessarily related to depression, but can be. Depression is quite common in the elderly. In contrast with younger patients who often respond to a cancer diagnosis with anxiety, depression is the more common disorder in older cancer patients. With proper support and medical attention, many of these patients can safely receive anticancer treatment.

Heart problems increase with age, and it is no surprise that older cancers patients have an increased risk of cardiac complications from intensive surgery, radiation, and chemotherapy (such as mitoxantrone). One should also keep in mind the cardiovascular complications that some hormonal therapies and chemotherapy (such as estramustine) can cause, especially blood clots (thrombosis).

Osteoporosis can be made worse by androgen deprivation therapy. This in turn, can result in fractures, falls, and progressive debility. Older men on hormonal therapy should have regular DEXA scans to monitor their bone health, and, when appropriate, take calcium and vitamin D supplements or bisphosphonates to minimize bone loss.

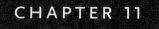

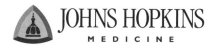

CHAPTER 11

JOHNS HOPKINS

M E D I C I N E

TRUSTED RESOURCES: FINDING ADDITIONAL INFORMATION ABOUT PROSTATE CANCER AND ITS TREATMENT

For many of you wanting to access more information about prostate cancer, a wealth of educational materials and resources is available from credible organizations. The following is a list of organizations, their means of access, and brief descriptions of services they provide. They may assist you further should you choose to seek additional help.

American Cancer Society

1-(800) ACS-2345 [227-2345]

www.cancer.org

This is a nationwide, community-based, voluntary health organization dedicated to eliminating cancer as a major health problem. Its mission is to prevent cancer, save lives, and diminish suffering from cancer through research, education, advocacy, and service.

American Prostate Society

(410) 859-3735

www.americanprostatesociety.com

This is a society established to provide support services for patients and family members affected by prostate cancer. The society provides ongoing, up-to-date information on benign and malignant prostate disorders.

American Foundation for Urologic Disease

(410) 689-3700

www.auafoundation.org

This organization is the nation's leading urologic health charity whose mission is to improve prevention, detection, and treatment, and ultimately to cure urologic diseases. The foundation is consolidated with the American Urological Association, thus integrating activities and programs of research, patient/public education, and patient advocacy through a foundation that is part of its medical specialty organization.

The Brady Urological Institute

(410) 955-6707

www.prostate.urol.jhu.edu

This organization refers to the group of dedicated physicians, scientists, and researchers in the Department of Urology at the Johns Hopkins Hospital whose mission is to continue developing and delivering state-of-the-art treatments and excellent clinical care for urological diseases. The Web site has many news articles about the latest research in prostate cancer performed at Johns Hopkins.

CaPCURE

1-(800) 757-CURE [757-2873]

www.capcure.org

This organization has a mission to find cures and controls for advanced prostate cancer. It is the leading, largest private source of funding for prostate cancer research in the world. CaPCURE is focused on moving research from the laboratory into the lives of patients. Its Web site may be accessed to learn updated information on recent research developments and clinical trials.

Hospice Foundation of America

(202) 638-5419

www.hospicefoundation.org

This organization provides leadership in the development and application of hospice and its philosophy of care. The foundation meets its mission by conducting programs of professional development, public education and information, research, publications, and health policy issues. It provides assistance for individual consumers of health care who are coping with issues of care giving, terminal illness, and grief.

National Cancer Institute
 1-(800) 4-CANCER [422-6237]
 www.cancer.gov

This component of the National Institutes of Health is the principal agency for cancer research and training of the U.S. government. Its mission is to disseminate new information about cancer research, education, and training while promoting the incorporation of state-of-the-art cancer treatments into clinical practice.

National Hospice and Palliative Care Organization
 1-(800) 658-8898
 (703) 837-1500
 www.nhpco.org

This organization is the largest nonprofit membership devoted exclusively to the promotion of hospice care in America. Its mission is advocacy for the rights of terminally ill persons. The organization provides informational and educational material for members while also providing information and referrals to the general public.

The National Prostate Cancer Coalition
 (202) 463-9455
 www.zerocancer.org

This organization is a major resource for reducing the burden of prostate cancer on American men and their families. Its activities involve awareness, outreach, and advocacy campaigns.

Prostate Cancer Foundation
1-(800) 757-CURE [757-2873]
www.prostatecancerfoundation.org

This foundation is the world's largest source of philanthropic support for prostate cancer research. Its primary mission is to fund promising research into better treatments and a cure for prostate cancer.

Us TOO International Prostate Cancer Education & Support Network
1-(800) 80-Us TOO [808-7866]
(630) 795-1002
www.ustoo.org

This is a grassroots organization started by prostate cancer survivors to serve prostate cancer survivors, their spouses/partners, and families. It is a not-for-profit charitable organization dedicated to communicating timely and reliable information that enables informed choices regarding detection and treatment of prostate cancer. The organization is represented by 325 support group chapters throughout the United States and the world.

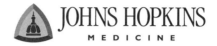

INFORMATION ABOUT
JOHNS HOPKINS

The James Buchanan Brady Urological Institute
The Johns Hopkins Hospital
  600 North Wolfe Street
  Baltimore, Maryland
  http://urology.jhu.edu/

The James Buchanan Brady Urological Institute at Johns Hopkins strives to remain the world leader in urology by delivering the finest patient care available, while simultaneously producing and translating revolutionary urological research for clinical application. The institute has developed a four-pronged approach for treating patients with urological cancer, which includes prevention, early detection, effective treatment of localized disease, and better ways to contain advanced disease. The institute's researchers are committed to discovering the genes that cause debilitating urological problems in children, and for uncovering the best treatments for men and women who experience urological complications.

About Johns Hopkins Medicine

Johns Hopkins Medicine unites physicians and scientists of the Johns Hopkins University School of Medicine with the organizations, health professionals, and facilities of the Johns Hopkins Health System. Its mission is to improve the health of the community and the world by setting the standard of excellence in medical education, research, and clinical care. Diverse and inclusive, Johns Hopkins Medicine has provided international leadership in the education of physicians and medical scientists in biomedical research and in the application of medical knowledge to sustain health since The Johns Hopkins Hospital opened in 1889.

If you plan to be evaluated or treated at Johns Hopkins, you will probably meet Dr. Burnett. He interacts with patients on a daily basis through evaluation, treatment planning, and management of prostate cancer.

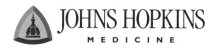

FURTHER READING

100 Questions & Answers About Prostate Cancer, Second Edition, Pamela Ellsworth, MD, Jones and Bartlett Publishers, 2009.

100 Questions & Answers About Prostate Disease, Kevin R. Loughlin, MD, and John Nimmo, Jones and Bartlett Publishers, 2007.

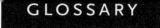

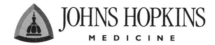

GLOSSARY

Adenocarcinoma: The most common form of prostate cancer.

Adjuvant systemic therapy: Treatment given after the primary treatment to increase the chances of a cure and treatment to prevent the cancer from recurring.

Alpha₁-antichymotrypsin: A circulating protein in the blood.

Anal sphincter: Rings of muscle at the opening of the anus.

Anal stricture: Often painful scar tissue at the anal sphincter.

Androgen deprivation therapy. *See* **Hormonal therapy.**

Anemia: Low red blood cell count.

Antiemetics: Antinausea medications.

Benign: Any tumor or growth which is not malignant or cancerous. A benign growth will not spread (or metastasize) to other areas of the body.

Benign prostatic enlargement: A noncancerous enlargement of the prostate.

Bilobar structure: A structure with two sides.

Biopsy: A procedure in which cells are collected for microscopic examination.

Bisphosphonates: A class of drugs that prevents the loss of bone mass.

Bladder neck contracture: Scar tissue at the bladder neck that causes narrowing.

Blood clots (thrombosis): Clumps that occur when the blood hardens from a liquid to a solid.

Bone scan: An X-ray that looks for signs of metastasis.

Brachytherapy: A form of internal radiation therapy.

CAT scan: Pictures of structures within the body created by a computer that takes the data from multiple X-ray images and turns them into pictures on a screen.

Cavernous nerves: Nerves responsible for penile erection.

Chemo brain: Difficulty with cognitive functioning as a side effect of receiving chemotherapy.

Chemotherapy: The use of chemical agents (drugs) to systemically treat cancer.

Clinical staging: Determination of the extent of disease based on clinical findings prior to any sort of treatment.

Clinical trial: A study of a drug or treatment with a large group of people testing the treatment.

Clinically significant erectile dysfunction: The inability to attain or sustain an erection for satisfactory sexual activity.

Clinically significant urinary incontinence: Loss of urinary control.

Cognitive impairment: Mental disorders distinguished by a limitation of mental functions (e.g., dementia).

Comorbidity: A disease or disorder someone already has prior to a new diagnosis.

Corticosteroids: Class of steroid hormones that are produced in the adrenal cortex.

Cryosurgery: The application of extreme cold to destroy abnormal or diseased tissue.

Dehydration: Occurs when the body does not have as much water and fluids as it should.

DEXA scan: Measures the density of bones.

Digital rectal examination: An assessment of whether a tumor is palpable by inserting a finger into the rectum.

Distant metastases: Cancer spread throughout the body.

Docetaxel: A chemotherapy drug given as treatment for some types of cancer.

Dorsiflexion exercises: Up and down movements of the feet when reclining in a chair or in bed.

External beam radiotherapy: Delivers radiation waves more focally and reduces the likelihood of radiation spread to structures beyond the prostate gland.

Erectile function: The inability to achieve erection.

Erythropoiesis: Stimulating agents such as epoetin (Procrit, Epogen) or darbepoetin (Aranesp).

Expectant management: Applied to patients who have a life expectancy of less than 10 years and for healthy men 65 years of age or older whose diagnostic workup suggests low-volume, low-grade prostate cancer ("watchful waiting").

Free PSA: A molecular form of PSA that is not bound to a circulating protein in the blood called alpha$_1$-antichymotrypsin.

Genetics counseling: Process by which patients or relatives are advised of the consequences and nature of the disorder, the probability of developing or transmitting it, and the options open to them.

Gleason score: A numerical grading system that defines the appearance of the cancerous tissue.

Grade: Aggressiveness level of the cancer.

Granulopoietic growth factors: Decrease the risk of infection.

Healthcare proxy: A document that permits a designated person to make decisions regarding your medical treatment when you are unable to do so.

High-intensity focused ultrasonography: Application of a heated beam of focused ultrasound waves guided to the prostate by an ultrasound probe placed into the rectum.

Hormonal therapy: Treatment that blocks the effects of hormones upon cancers that depend on hormones to grow.

Hospice/palliative care: Such services help in preparing for one's leaving this world, dying with dignity as well as with pain under control, and having emotional needs of the loved one's family met.

Interstitial seed (brachytherapy) radiotherapy: Surgical placement of radiated seeds, such as radioactive iodine-125 or palladium-102 seeds, into the prostate.

Laparoscopic approach: Surgery involving multiple stab-like incisions for passage of instruments.

Living will: A document that outlines what care you want in the event you become unable to communicate due to coma or heavy sedation.

Lymph node: Tissue in the lymphatic system that filter lymph fluid and help the immune system fight disease.

Malignant: Cancerous; growing rapidly and out of control.

Medical oncologist: A cancer specialist who helps determine treatment choices.

Metastis: The process by which cancer spreads from the place at which it first arose as a primary tumor to distant locations in the body.

MRI: A medical imaging technique most commonly used in radiology to visualize the internal structure and function of the body.

Mucositis: Mouth sores.

Myelosuppression: Low white blood cell count.

Nerve-sparing: Technique for protecting the erection-producing nerves surrounding the prostate during prostate cancer surgery.

Neurotoxicity: Adverse effects on the structure or function of the central and/or peripheral nervous system caused by exposure to a toxic chemical.

Nomogram: Provides information regarding whether the disease is contained to the prostate gland, spread locally beyond the prostate gland, or spread distantly into lymph node tissue or elsewhere.

Oncology nurses: Nurses in this field provide care and support for patients diagnosed with cancer. They are responsible for administering chemotherapy and managing symptoms related to cancer illnesses.

Open retropubic approach: Surgery involving usually one small incision at the low abdomen.

Orchiectomy: Surgical procedure to remove the testicles from the scrotum.

Osteoporosis: A disease of bone that leads to an increased risk of fracture.

Palliative management: Care to relieve the symptoms of cancer and to keep the best quality of life for as long as possible without seeking to cure cancer.

Palpable: Whether hardness or a nodule is felt with the finger inserted into the rectum and placed on the prostate.

Pathological staging: Extent of cancer found in surgically removed tissue.

Pathologist: A specialist trained to distinguish normal from abnormal cells.

Pelvic CAT scan: *See* CAT scan.

Pelvic MRI study: Frequently obtained for clinical staging and may be most relevant for many radiation therapy recommendations.

Penile atrophy: Changes in the dimensions and structure of the penis.

Perineal approach: Surgery involving usually one small incision.

Peripheral neuropathy: Nerve damage from, e.g., diabetes.

Preoperative tests: Tests are done to ensure that there are no acute health conditions requiring attention prior to undergoing surgery or radiation.

Prostascint scan: Used to check for lymph node invasion in men with prostate cancer.

Prostate biopsy: Diagnostic technique for prostate cancer in which a needle instrument is used to sample multiple prostate pieces (usually 12) for pathological assessment.

Prostate cancer: The presence of malignant cells in the prostate.

Prostate cancer surgeon: A urologic surgeon with surgical expertise in performing radical prostatectomy, the removal of the prostate, appropriate surrounding tissue, and pelvic lymph nodes.

Prostate imaging radiologist: *See* **Radiologist.**

Prostate pathologist: *See* **Pathologist.**

Prostate-specific antigen (PSA) level: The amount of prostate-specific antigen in the blood.

Prostatitis: Inflammation of the prostate gland.

PSA density: A determination of PSA value adjusted for prostate size.

PSA monitoring: Monitoring changes in PSA level over time.

PSA velocity: The rate of change in PSA over time.

Psychosocial support staff: Staff who assist in coping with stress associated with diagnosis through recovery and beyond.

Pulmonary embolism: Caused by blood clots that form in the lower legs after surgery and then become dislodged and circulate to the lungs.

Radiation oncologist: A cancer specialist who determines the amount of radiation therapy required.

Radiation therapy: Use of high-energy X-rays to kill cancer cells and shrink tumors.

Radical prostatectomy: Surgical removal of the entire prostate.

Radical prostatectomy with bilateral pelvic lymph node dissection: Surgical removal of the entire prostate, along with pelvic lymph nodes.

Radiologist: A physician specializing in the treatment of disease using radiation therapy.

Risk profile: Outline of risk factors related to prostate cancer.

Salvage radiation therapy: Used in patients with rising PSA after radical prostatectomy.

Salvage radical prostatectomy: Used in patients with recurring prostate cancer, usually after radiation therapy.

Secondary prevention: Process to reduce the recurrence of prostate cancer after initial treatment.

Seminal vesicles: Either of a pair of pouchlike glands situated on each side of the male urinary bladder that secrete seminal fluid and nourish and promote the movement of spermatozoa through the urethra.

Serial PSA testing: Testing of PSA levels over a period of time.

Side effects: Problems that occur in addition to the desired therapeutic effect.

Social worker: This professional is involved in support issues surrounding the management of prostate cancer and also in addressing financial concerns that arise surrounding clinical management.

Sonographic volume: Size of an organ or structure based on measurements using ultrasound waveforms.

Stage: A numerical determination of how far the cancer has progressed.

Surgery: Measures that are concerned with diseases and conditions that require or are amenable to operative procedures.

Surgical margin: Visible normal tissue removed with surgical excision of a tumor.

Survivor volunteer: This individual "who has been there before" offers tremendous emotional support and complements the service the professional staff provides.

Testosterone: A male hormone.

Thrombosis: *See* **Blood clots**.

Transrectal ultrasonography: This test uses a small rectal probe to create an image of the prostate gland.

Transurethral resection: A procedure in which an instrument is inserted through the penis to scrape out cancerous tissue interfering with urination.

Tumor: Mass or lump of extra tissue.

Ureters: Tube-like structures that carry urine from the kidneys down to the bladder on each side of the pelvis.

Urinary control: Ability to control the voiding of urine.

Urinary frequency: Urinating at frequent intervals during the day or with nighttime sleep.

Urinary sphincter: Muscles used to control the flow of urine from the urinary bladder.

Urinary urgency: The inability to suppress the sensation to urinate.

Urologic surgeon: A physician who specializes in the medical and surgical treatment of diseases of the genital (in males) and urinary tracts.

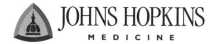

Index